DYSFUNCTIONAL BEHAVIOUR
IN DEMENTIA:
A CLINICIAN'S GUIDE

The essential guide for clinicians who care for people with dementia

- Understand how dysfunctional behaviour fits into the overall picture of dementia
- Learn practical management tools and techniques
- Develop skills in non-pharmacological approaches as well as drug therapy
- Easy-to-use clinical tools, key-point summaries and case studies for rapid learning

M. O'Donnell
D.W. Molloy
K. Rabheru

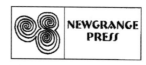

NEWGRANGE PRESS

First Edition, 2001

ISBN: 0-9688010-7-2

1. A clinicians guide to the management of Dysfunctional behaviour in dementia
2. Dementia
3. Psychosis

Published in 2001 by Newgrange Press

Newgrange Press (Canada),
Orkney House,
428 Orkney Road,
RR1 Troy,
Ontario L0R 2B0
Canada

Telephone: (905) 628-0354, Fax: (905) 628-4901
Email: idecide@netcom.ca
Website:www.newgrangepress.com

PRINTED IN CANADA
by *Artco Graphics Inc.*

DYSFUNCTIONAL BEHAVIOUR IN DEMENTIA

Dr. M. O'Donnell
Dr. D.W. Molloy
Dr. K. Rabheru

Editorial Board

Dr. Stefan Krajcik MD. PhD., Head of Geriatric Department, Slovak Postgraduate Academy of Medicine, National Institute of TB and Respiratory Diseases, Krajinska, Bratislava, Slovakia.

Judy Lever RN BSc. MSc., Nurse Clinician in Geriatrics, Geriatric Research Group, McMaster University, Hamilton, Ontario, Canada.

Dr. Eric Mohr PhD. RPsych, Chairman and Chief Executive Officer, Professor of Medicine and Psychology, CroMedica Group of Medicines Development Companies, Victoria, British Columbia, Canada.

Dr. James O' Brien MD., The Margaret D. Smock Endowed Professor of Geriatrics in the Department of Family and Community Medicine, University of Louisville, Kentucky, U.S.A.

Dr. Des O'Neill MB FRCPI, Consultant Geriatrician, Health Adelaide Hospitals, Trinity College, Dublin, Ireland.

Dr. Kenneth Rockwood MD FRCPC, Professor of Geriatric Medicine, Dalhousie University, Halifax, Nova Scotia, Canada.

Glenda Smith Dip Psych Nurse RN, Clinical Consultant for Longterm Care, Psychiatric Consulting Service, Capital Health,Edmonton, Alberta, Canada.

Dr. David Strang MB FRCPC, Consultant Geriatrician, Assistant Professor, University of Manitoba, Winnipeg, Manitoba, Canada.

Dr. John Tooth MB FRANZCP Geriatric Psychiatry, Medical Director, ADARDS Nursing Home, Tasmania 7054, Australia.

Dr. Irene Tuttle MB BCh., Family Doctor, Geriatric Research Group, McMaster University, Ontario, Canada.

This book is dedicated to
Dr. Michael Hyland,
a gentleman and a scholar.

TABLE OF CONTENTS

Chapter 1

WHY IS THIS BOOK NEEDED?

About 2 to 3% of people between the ages of 65 and 75 years have dementia. The prevalence increases exponentially thereafter, reaching about 40% by the tenth decade[1]. In the next few decades the prevalence of dementia will triple as the population ages.

Alzheimer's disease is the most common cause of dementia in the elderly, accounting for approximately 65% of cases. Other less common causes include Lewy body dementia, Vascular Dementia, Parkinson's disease with dementia and Frontotemporal dementia. Early, accurate diagnosis is essential as treatment options vary depending on the clinical type and stage.[2]

The most obvious feature of dementia is **dysfunctional behaviour in dementia (DBD)**, defined as **an inappropriate action or response, other than an activity of daily living, in a given social milieu that is a problem for the caregiver or patient.** DBD is an active demonstration of the person's inability to cope with his or her environment.

While previously thought to be more common in the later stages, DBD develops early in the disease, sometimes even before cognitive decline is apparent, and tends to increase in frequency and severity as the disease progresses.

DBD puts more burden on caregivers than deficits in activities of daily living (ADL), depression and cognitive impairment combined.[3,4] DBD is the most common reason for institutionalization of demented patients because caregivers burn out and give up when they are unable to manage these problems.[4,5] If clinicians do not describe, assess, and manage DBD in a timely and effective manner, caregivers will burn out, and patients will be institutionalized prematurely.

To date, DBD has received less attention than the cognitive or functional aspects of dementia. Lack of consensus and guidelines for the assessment and management of DBD has led to inconsistency in diagnosis and treatment. Patients who have behavioural problems are more likely to receive pharmacological and/or physical restraints, resulting in further humiliation, loss of autonomy, frustration and immobility, and increased morbidity and mortality. This is regrettable, because DBD may be more responsive to treatment than any other domain in dementia. There are a variety of interventions that effectively manage and resolve DBD, thereby improving caregivers' and patients' quality of life.

The recent expansion in our understanding and treatment of dementia and its related disorders, including DBD, has led to a more active and focused approach to assessment, diagnosis and treatment. Clinicians need to recognize DBD, assess it comprehensively, develop a care plan and score the effectiveness of the treatment strategies employed. Inadequate assessment and/or management of DBD results in excessive morbidity and mortality among patients and caregivers[6] with unnecessary use of health care services.

Reported prevalence rates for DBD vary in the literature because of inconsistency in the definitions and instruments used, and in cohorts studied (community versus institutionalized patients). As a starting point, a simple clinical nomenclature and classification of DBD is essential for reliable and valid interpretation, reporting and documentation.

It is our intention in this book to provide health care workers who care for patients with dementia with a comprehensive and practical guide to DBD. We have performed comprehensive reviews of the literature on this challenging topic and have attempted to develop a clear and practical approach for clinicians. In order to obtain and provide consensus, we have sought input from our editorial board, a group of respected, dedicated and esteemed clinicians. They have acted as a sounding board and provided us with careful, thoughtful and thorough feedback. Their input has significantly improved the text and we are sincerely grateful to them for their time, expertise and support. We would like to especially thank Dr. Ken Rockwood for his generous and insightful input in developing the goals of treatment. Special thanks to Helen Byrt for her editorial assistance. Thanks also to Art & Sheri Cabeceira for their time and expertise in the development and production of this book.

We would like to acknowledge and thank our local branch of the Alzheimer's Society, who provide enormous support and assistance to us in our work. We recommend that every caregiver who has to deal with dementia should be encouraged to contact their local Alzheimer's Society to learn more about the disease, access educational resourses and/or join a caregiver support group.

Chapter 2

DEMENTIA OVERVIEW

Dementia is defined as **a group of brain disorders that affect multiple cognitive functions, such as memory, language, visuospatial perception, praxis, insight, reasoning and judgment.**

Dementia, like schizophrenia, can be described as having "negative" (lost) and "positive" (new) clinical features.

The main negative features are impairments in cognition, mood, and the ability to perform activities of daily living (ADL). There is progressive impairment in instrumental ADL (IADL) such as driving, shopping, cooking and managing finances. Later, impairments occur in basic ADL (BADL), such as washing, bathing, toileting, feeding and walking. Cognitive loss impairs the ability to learn new information (disorientation to time and place), and also results in impaired short-term memory (confusion and disorientation); **agnosia** (inability to recognize faces or objects); **anomia** (inability to name objects); **apraxia** (inability to perform learned tasks); **aphasia** (inability to find words and communicate needs); and **acalculia** (inability to use numbers). These disabling losses, which make the affected individual increasingly vulnerable to physical illness, depression and death, place a tremendous burden on caregivers.

These progressive deficits can be categorized into an "ABCDE of dementia"—five major domains that impact on social and occupational functioning (see also Fig. 1.1)—as follows:

- ADL—the ability to perform activities of daily living independently.
- Behaviour—the emergence of a wide constellation of dysfunctional behaviours.
- Cognitive impairment—with memory loss, and progressive aphasia, agnosia, apraxia and deficits in a wide variety of cognitive domains.
- Depression—negative alteration in mood with accompanying vegetative signs, e.g., sleep, energy, appetite, etc.
- Effect on caregiver—increased physical, emotional, social and psychological burden on family and friends who care for people with dementia.

Assessment of a patient with dementia is not a simple matter, and the differential diagnosis of dementia is complex (see Table 4.1). In our own outpatients' clinic we use this "ABCDE" as a clinical tool/checklist to focus each assessment and ensure that it covers all the domains of this complex group of disorders that are covered in Chapters 5 and 9.

Chapter 3

DYSFUNCTIONAL BEHAVIOUR IN DEMENTIA

"We have no sooner started than Iris is jumping up and down in agitation. Where are we going? Where is the bus taking us? She won't sit down but rushes to the front...before I can stop her she is speaking agitatedly to the bus driver...I apologise to the driver, who remains ominously silent."

—*John Bailey, in "Iris: A Memoir of Iris Murdoch"*

Learning Objectives:
- Understand features, aetiology, causes and prevalence of dysfunctional behaviour in dementia (DBD).
- Consider causative theories and appreciate that they are not mutually exclusive.
- Develop an analytical approach to DBD by classifying it into four distinct categories of dysfunctional behaviour: repetitions, responses (external - caregiver directed and internal - patient distress), activities and perceptions.

OVERVIEW OF DYSFUNCTIONAL BEHAVIOUR IN DEMENTIA

Dysfunctional behaviour in dementia can be defined as **an inappropriate action or response, other than an activity of daily living, in a given social milieu, that is a problem for the caregiver or patient.**

It should be emphasized that the behaviour must be problematic before it is deemed dysfunctional. Usually, the more unpredictable, disruptive and inappropriate the behaviour, the greater the challenge for caregivers. DBD includes a wide variety of behaviours, ranging from benign repetitive activities to overt physical aggression. Figure 3.2 provides a simple nomenclature and classification of the cluster of symptoms and signs that are included in DBD.

How each person behaves is determined by numerous variables including personality, mood, general wellbeing, intelligence, education, social background, environment, needs and so on (see Fig. 3.1). DBD includes any dysfunctional behaviour occurring in the setting of a dementing illness that may be exacerbated by a variety of factors, such as psychiatric disorders, inappropriate responses from caregivers, unsuitable environment and medical problems (pain, fecal impaction, hunger, dehydration or delirium).

Dysfunctional behaviour is a visible manifestation of the patient's frustration, anxiety, depression and/or inability to cope, in the face of changes in these environmental factors.

Figure 3.1. Factors that contribute to DBD

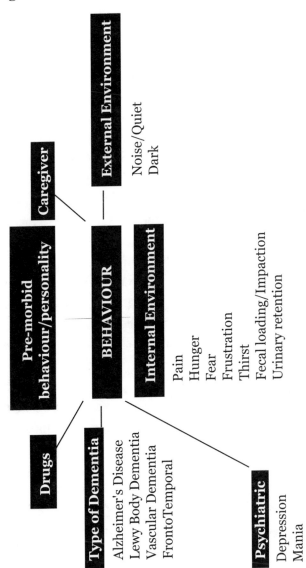

It does not take much imagination to realize that DBD is more distressing and puts more pressure on caregivers than cognitive decline, depression and the inability to perform activities of daily living (ADL).[1,2] DBD is the most common reason for institutionalization in dementia, as caregivers burn out and give up the struggle to cope.[2,4]

There is now a growing recognition that both patients and caregivers can be helped by a combination of environmental, behavioural and pharmacological interventions. Our understanding of dementia and DBD has expanded in recent years, leading to the development of a more active and focused approach to assessment, diagnosis and treatment.

Environmental factors are central to management because they have a large bearing on what is considered to be normal or abnormal behaviour in any given setting. For example, shouting at the top of one's voice may be considered normal at a sporting event, but dysfunctional in the home. DBD is the manifestation of a patient's responses to his or her environment, and his or her attempts to cope with it. Chapter 6 outlines how these considerations can be used in an environmental approach to the management of DBD.

The recent development of "atypical" antipsychotics, and their use in the treatment of DBD, represents a significant advance in pharmacological management.

"Traditional" antipsychotics have serious side-effect profiles, especially when used as maintenance therapy. Antipsychotics can be used for months, even years, in dementia, so most patients develop extrapyramidal effects (rigidity, tremor and bradykinesia) that reduce mobility and increase the risk of falls. These extrapyramidal side effects can have a devastating effect on patients' occupational and social functioning. For this reason, traditional antipsychotics are only recommended as parenteral short-term medications in emergency situations. Treatments that avoid these side effects are a significant clinical advance.

Atypical antipsychotics produce fewer undesirable side effects such as extrapyramidal bradykinesia, dystonia, tremor, dyskinesia and akathisia, without compromising treatment efficacy. The atypicals also have fewer anticholinergic effects such as confusion, sedation, dry mouth, urinary retention and/or constipation.

For a detailed review of pharmacological management of DBD, see Chapter 7.

AETIOLOGY AND PREVALENCE

While the exact aetiology and dynamics at play in DBD are often uncertain, it is certain that DBD is an inevitable consequence of cognitive decline. The prevalence of DBD in Alzheimer's disease (AD) ranges from approximately 60% at home to 90% in institutionalized older adults[10] . The prevalence varies depending on definitions used to describe behavioural dysfunction. Most patients who develop DBD will continue to have symptoms for the rest of their lives.

The prevalence of DBD is equally as high in patients with frontotemporal dementia, Lewy body dementia and vascular dementia. Each dementia has its own characteristic constellation of behaviour patterns. For example, AD typically presents with repetitive behaviours because of short-term memory loss. Lewy body dementia presents with hallucinations and systematized delusions, while patients with frontotemporal dementia characteristically have disinhibition, hyperorality, loss of social graces and impulsivity or apathy. People with vascular dementia are more likely to have aggression, depression and anxiety.

CAUSATIVE MODELS OF DBD

There are many theories about the causes of DBD and about why certain types of dementia display different patterns and constellations of behavioural symptoms. These causative models are not mutually exclusive and it is likely that DBD has a wide variety of contributing causes. For each patient you need to consider all of these models in your assessment.

Diminished Adaptive Capacity Model[3]
Dementia causes a reduction in functional ability, usually manifesting as impairment in activities of

daily living (ADL). This loss of independence results in frustration and is compounded by the inability to express concerns and feelings such as anxiety, loneliness, grief and loss. As independence diminishes and limitations increase, there is more and more disruption in responses, reactions, perception and routines with increasing inability to cope.

Even relatively minor stresses, such as intercurrent illnesses or subtle changes in environment, together with this reduced ability to interpret and communicate, can cause problems to escalate with increased morbidity—even mortality.

Stress Model [3]

Even relatively minor challenges that require simple problem-solving create greater stress in people with dementia. People with dementia are more prone to social, psychological, emotional and health stresses, making their inability to interpret, understand, assimilate and formulate appropriate responses to alterations in their environment more pronounced. Loss of autonomy, social skills and acumen, along with growing social isolation, contribute to these difficulties. Inability to assess and integrate change, combined with a reduced capacity to cope with these stresses, provoke inappropriate responses, i.e., DBD.

Characterologic Model[5,6]

From early childhood, people learn to use behaviour-modifying strategies to cope with hassles and irritations without showing overt signs of frustration or anger. "Normal" behaviour is contextual and learning evolves over time. What is considered normal is different for babies, toddlers, teenagers and adults. It is modified by context, environment, culture and individual goals and needs. Dementia may accentuate the underlying personality traits and character of the person. The person becomes less flexible, responsive and amenable to change.

In dementia, it is important to re-define what is "normal" behaviour. Patients' cognitive processing is damaged and they are more vulnerable to new stresses; they cannot interpret changes in the environment, learn, or adapt appropriately. Normal responses are not possible, rendering patients more susceptible to having their actions labelled as "inappropriate responses," which we call DBD.

The "premorbid personality" may affect the type and severity of DBD. For example, people with fussy, controlling personalities are more likely to develop obsessive behaviours. In theory, people with aggressive, pushy, domineering personalities might become aggressive; however, studies have failed to demonstrate such a correlation.[6] Behaviour is not always attributable to dementia and people who were verbally and/or physically aggressive prior to the onset of dementia, are likely to continue as the disease unmasks or exacerbates these established behaviours.

Neurobiologic Model [7,8,9]

This model suggests that specific deficiencies in neurotransmitters are associated with certain behaviour patterns. For example, serotonin deficiency contributes to depression. In dementia, differential neurochemical deficiencies or combinations thereof, particularly in acetylcholine, serotonin and noradrenaline, may account for particular behaviours. This model has received research emphasis because it may lead to specific, targeted, therapeutic interventions that restore the balance in neurotransmitters, thereby alleviating particular behaviours. While cholinergic drugs may alleviate some dysfunctional behaviours, it is not clear if this improvement in DBD results solely from the drugs' effects on cognition, or whether cholinergic drugs have independent effects on DBD. Functional defects in certain portions of the brain have been correlated with the presence of psychotic symptoms in Alzheimer's disease.[8]

As cognitive impairment increases, the prevalence and severity of DBD grows. As individuals become more impaired, adaptive strategies are overwhelmed, coping mechanisms fail, stress increases, and neurotransmitter levels drop as the neuropathology progresses. Dementia promotes and increases stress, while impairing the individual's ability to cope, against a backdrop of progressive structural and chemical abnormalities in the brain.

CLASSIFICATION OF DYSFUNCTIONAL BEHAVIOURS

Dysfunctional behaviour in dementia includes a wide variety of different behaviours and, characteristically, patients have many. The persistence, unpredictability and variety of the behaviours, combined with a lack of response to reasoning or traditional behaviour-modification, add to the caregiver's burden.

At present there are a variety of different terms used for these different behaviours, such as **Behavioural and Psychological Symptoms of Dementia (BPSD)**. In this book, we use the term **Dysfunctional Behaviour in Dementia (DBD)**.

Classification of these behaviours is not an easy matter. Consider a person who resists care by pushing a caregiver away: this could be called aggression, anger, agitation, resisting care, acting out, striking out, or a normal response of a confused older adult who does not understand the caregiver's intentions.

We have attempted to simplify the nomenclature of these different behaviours by grouping them into four categories in a user-friendly fashion, to facilitate screening, assessment, diagnosis, treatment and measurement of response to treatment (see Fig. 3.2). Accurate assessment and diagnosis helps caregivers to understand, interpret and manage these behaviours. Of course, we recognize that there is some overlap among these categories, but we have nonetheless attempted to simplify the nomenclature and classification to facilitate a more structured and focused approach to assessment and management.

The four categories are as follows:

1. **Dysfunctional Repetitions**
2. **Dysfunctional Responses :**
   Internal (patient distress) and
   External (caregiver directed)
3. **Dysfunctional Activities**
4. **Dysfunctional Perceptions.**

Each category contains a number of specific dysfunctional behaviours. Aggression and agitation are by far the most problematic behaviours, and caregivers exposed to these behaviours frequently give up, burn out and institutionalize the patients.

Figure 3.2. Simple nomenclature and
classification of DBD

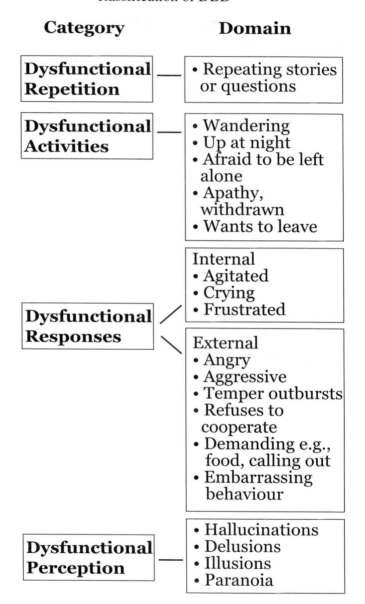

<u>Dysfunctional Repetitions</u>

Repetitive behaviour includes stories or questions that are repeated for no apparent purpose, or repeated actions (like dressing and undressing, hand-washing, etc.).

1. <u>Dysfunctional Responses</u>

A. *External response (Caregiver-directed)*

A dysfunctional external response is any action that is directed at another and includes a variety of different behaviours that are repeated, inappropriate and put the patient and/or caregiver at risk.

This category deals with responses of patients to caregivers, whereas dysfunctional activities (see below) deals with disruption in routines and may not be directed at caregivers, e.g., up at night, wandering.

Responses are usually directed towards a caregiver, e.g., aggression, shouting, demanding. They may result when the caregiver wants the person to do something, e.g., get dressed, or when the patient demands something from the caregiver.

This category includes the following:

Anger

Caregivers may interpret a whole range of responses as anger, e.g., tone of voice, physical gestures, etc.

Aggression

Includes physical gestures such as fist waving or motor activity directed towards others that may harm them, e.g., striking out, pushing, hitting, punching, kicking, biting or verbal aggression, which includes shouting, threatening or swearing.

Temper Outbursts

Habitual, sudden displays of anger or loss of composure, and/or petulance.

Demanding Behaviour

Repeatedly insisting of caregivers in a forceful way, often in spite of repeated refusals, e.g., demanding food despite having just eaten, calling out.

Refusal to Co-operate

Lack of co-operation while performing tasks or other activities.

Embarrassing Behaviour in Public

Can take a variety of forms, e.g., inappropriate sexual demands, actions or abusive comments.

B. Dysfunctional Internal Responses (Patient Distress)

This category includes non-specific responses usually not directed at others. These are behaviours usually observed by caregivers where patients suffer because of their inability to cope with their environment and include the following:

Agitation

Disturbed, excited behaviour with mental anxiety or concern, e.g., pacing.

Crying

Sobbing, moaning, wailing or any audible or visible expression of sadness, grief or regret.

Frustration

Discontent because of inability to achieve desires or needs.

3. Dysfunctional Activities

Wandering

Walking or moving about while disoriented to place.

Up at Night

Includes any type of sleep disturbance, such as insomnia (decreased sleep), hypersomnia (increased sleep), and changes or disruption in sleep/wake patterns with frequent nocturnal waking. Patients commonly nap during the day and are awake at night.

Afraid to be Left Alone

This is the most common phobia in dementia. A phobia is a persistent, irrational, exaggerated and pathological dread of some specific stimulus, resulting in a compelling desire to avoid it.

Patients follow caregivers around the house like

puppies or toddlers. Caregivers describe patients as "a noose around their neck" or "shadows" because they can follow them from room to room, even into the bathroom, and may refuse to allow other caregivers into the house. These patients are often unable to perform or sustain activities alone. Caregivers subjected to this behaviour feel a complete loss of privacy.

Withdrawal

Includes apathy, with dulled emotional tone, associated with detachment or indifference. Apathy is included in this category because it usually manifests as withdrawal from daily activities and is its most prominent feature. It may also be considered a dysfunctional response.

Wanting to Leave

Occurs when the patient wants to "go home to mother and father" or "collect the children" or "go to work." They are often living in a period of life that has passed and are usually disoriented to place and time.

4. <u>Dysfunctional Perceptions</u>

Hallucinations

False sensory perceptions not associated with real external stimuli. May be visual (sight), auditory (hearing), olfactory (smell) or tactile (touch).

Illusions

Misinterpretations of reality. For example, a person with dementia may think that television characters are real and in the room at home or that a rake on the ground is a snake.

Delusions (including Paranoia)

False beliefs that something is real that is not, that is not consistent with the person's intelligence or cultural background, and cannot be corrected by reasoning. Common beliefs are that a relative is a stranger, and that people are stealing things or trying to cause harm.

Hoarding/Hiding

Collecting, storing or hiding objects in a "safe" place or places.

Others

Includes behaviours that are not included in the above listing because they may present in a bizarre or unusual way. Examples would be refusing to change clothes, urinating inappropriately or some rituals that have no apparent purpose.

CLINICAL GEMS

- There is no single causative theory for DBD. It involves an interplay of numerous psychological and physical (neurobiological) dynamics.
- DBD occurs in most people with dementia.
- Most patients with DBD will have it for the rest of their lives; therefore, goals of treatment should be realistic and geared towards reducing and controlling symptoms.
- DBD affects two groups of people: the demented person and the caregiver.
- There are four categories of DBD: Dysfunctional repetitions, responses, activities and perceptions.
- Each of these dysfunctional categories of behaviour require different approaches to treatment.

Chapter 4

PATTERNS OF DBD IN DIFFERENT DEMENTIAS[1-10]

"Ambrose came out of the kitchen one night, frowning. Everyone laughed because he was carrying the toaster oven and they thought he was going to use it as a prop for one of his famous jokes . . . But that night he looked at Peggy. 'I've forgotten how to make the tea.'"

—*Sandra Sabatini, "The One With the News."*

Learning Objectives:

- Understand the common causes of dementia.
  Be able to review the common patterns of
  dysfunctional behaviour in dementia (DBD)
  that accompany each type of dementia and
  learn how this assists with diagnosis.
- Differentiate between depression
  (pseudodementia) and dementia.
- Differentiate between delirium and dementia.

INTRODUCTION

There are over 60 causes of dementia. **Alzheimer's disease** (AD) accounts for over 60 percent of cases, followed by **vascular dementia** (VD) and **Lewy body dementia** (LBD), which together account for about 30% of the remaining causes. Lewy body dementia has been increasingly recognized in recent years. Often there is a combination of causes (**mixed dementia**); for example, a patient with a brain scan indicative of multi-infarct may also have AD. Up to 60% of patients with Parkinson's disease have AD pathology and up to 28% of patients with clinically diagnosed AD have Lewy bodies[1]. Each disease has certain distinctive profiles (see Table 3.1).

In AD, short-term memory loss is the most common presenting complaint and reason for assessment. If asked, caregivers will report that changes in behaviour occurred even before the memory loss became apparent; for example, a caregiver may notice memory loss because the patient repeats questions or stories. Thus, DBD is a common clinical presentation of memory loss.

In some dementias, such as frontotemporal dementia (FTD) or Lewy body dementia, DBD can be the presenting complaint even before memory loss becomes an issue. The sequence, pattern and severity of DBD provide important clues to the underlying diagnosis.

Alzheimer's disease, vascular dementia, Lewy body dementia and frontotemporal dementia each have characteristic patterns of DBD at onset and as the disease progresses. However, as each disease progresses into the later stages and disability increases, they all start to look the same and share a single common clinical pathway in the end.

A summary of the differential diagnosis of dementia is presented in Table 4.1. Rare causes of dementia are presented in Table 4.2.

ALZHEIMER'S DISEASE

In 1901, Dr Alois Alzheimer first described the case of Auguste D., who presented with florid behavioural problems, including paranoid delusions, auditory hallucinations, wandering, and agitation with outbursts of screaming. Brain pathology revealed neurofibrillary tanges and neuritic plaques.

The most common presenting DBD in Alzheimer's disease is repeating questions and repeating stories. The natural history of behavioural dysfunction in AD is less predictable than that of cognitive decline.

The history of short-term memory loss in AD classically has two cardinal features. The first is an insidious onset with gradual progression over years. The second feature is that the rate of memory loss accelerates over time. Caregivers will say, "he's had it for three years, but we've noticed a sharper decline in the last six months than in the previous three years. It's getting worse recently and is much more noticeable in the past few months."

With progressive cognitive decline, DBD becomes more florid and severe. In the middle stages of AD, patients develop delusions, hallucinations and/ or misperceptions of reality. When they look in mirrors and do not recognize themselves, or do not recognize family members, they think that "there are strangers in the house." They do not see people or objects that are **not** there; rather, they misinterpret or fail to recognize the objects and people that **are** there. This is **agnosia** (failure to recognize familiar faces or objects) that accompanies the **amnesia** (memory loss).

Patients with AD exhibit gender differences in behaviour patterns. Men are more likely to exhibit apathy and pacing whereas women are more likely to have abnormal eating and sleeping.[2] Our clinical experience has been that men with Alzheimer's disease are more likely to exhibit anger, aggression and embarrassing behaviour whereas crying and hiding things is more common in women.

LEWY BODY DEMENTIA[1,4]

First described in 1923 by Friedrich H. Lewy, Lewy body dementia accounts for approximately 15 to 25% of all cases of dementia[4], making it the second or third most common dementia. We have discussed it in detail as it has achieved recent clinical prominence and because it is a diagnosis that is often overlooked.

Histologically, diagnostic eosinophilic Lewy bodies (surrogate markers of neuronal loss) occur throughout the brain and cause a variety of presentations and clinical patterns, depending on the location and severity of lesions. Lewy bodies in the nigrostriatal area cause the characteristic movement disorder of Parkinson's disease. In the autonomic ganglia, they are associated with postural hypotension. Cognitive impairment and psychosis are typically associated with limbic cortical and neocortical involvement.

Lewy bodies have been found in as many as 28% of brains of people with AD[1]. Although definitive diagnosis of any dementia can only be made at autopsy, clinical diagnostic criteria have been developed to assist with clinical diagnosis. The International Consensus Criteria[4] focus on three cardinal features (see below). If two of these features are present, the diagnosis is **probable Lewy body dementia**. If one is present, the diagnosis is **possible Lewy body dementia**.

1. Fluctuating level of confusion

This can be a difficult feature to discern on history and is very often a retrospective observation. AD patients tend to become more confused in the evening (**sundowning**), after sleep or during the night when they awake. By contrast, the fluctuating pattern with Lewy body dementia is less predictable. Some caregivers will describe intermittent confusion, e.g., hallucinations, coming on infrequently (every month or so) and lasting for minutes or hours. Over time these episodes become more frequent (every few days or weeks) and last longer, e.g., for 2 to 3 days or even more. Eventually, they never seem to go away. When they are confused, patients mumble, see things or talk to people who are not there.

2. Visual hallucinations

AD patients see themselves in the mirror and think that there is a stranger in the house. People with AD talk to photographs and people on television. Delusions tend to be superficial, i.e., "there is someone else in the house." This is better classified as a misperception than a "real" hallucination. In Lewy body dementia, patients describe the hallucinations in greater detail. They see children or animals, think that their daughter is still living upstairs and/or talk to people sitting in empty chairs. These hallucinations may not disturb patients or they may complain that the person "who was here today would not speak to me".

Patients can describe hallucinations better in Lewy body dementia because the hallucinations appear earlier in the disease when patients still have the language skills to describe them. In AD the "hallucinations" or misperceptions appear in the middle stages when SMMSE (Standardized Mini Mental State Examination) [11] scores are in the teens (10 to 20) and the patient may not have the vocabulary, memory or communication skills to describe them. By contrast, in Lewy body dementia patients often **present** with visual hallucinations when the SMMSE scores are still almost normal (24 or more). These patients not only have the cognitive capacity to describe what they see, but many even understand that these are hallucinations.

3. Spontaneous Parkinsonism

Classically, the clinical triad of bradykinesia, rigidity and resting tremor need to be clinically sought, as these signs may be early, mild and subtle. In Lewy body dementia, the negative symptoms of bradykinesia and rigidity are more frequent, and the positive feature, tremor, is uncommon.

Other supporting features of Lewy body dementia include the following:
- Sensitivity to antipsychotics
- Repeated falls
- Syncope
- Transient loss of consciousness

- Systematized delusions
- Auditory, tactile or olfactory hallucinations.

A diagnosis of Lewy body dementia is less likely in the presence of stroke, or if there is evidence of other causes of cognitive impairment that are more likely to account for these features. It is important to exclude Lewy body dementia before a diagnosis of Alzheimer's disease is made. In particular, exclude the diagnosis of Lewy body dementia in elderly patients who present with delirium, movement disorders or falls. Because of the variety of possible presentations of DBD, patients may present to a variety of different services including geriatrics (memory loss), neurology, internal medicine (falls or syncope) or psychiatry (delusions and hallucinations).

An important diagnostic feature of Lewy body dementia is the onset and pattern of DBD, and its relationship to cognitive impairment. One is often surprised to find that in spite of delusions, visual hallucinations, and physical disability from bradykinesia and rigidity, these patients score higher than expected on the SMMSE because cognition is relatively well preserved at presentation.

Another important diagnostic clue to Lewy body dementia is the early loss of spatial orientation, demonstrated by failure to reproduce the two five-sided figures on the SMMSE. This may even be the first deficit seen. AD patients typically don't lose spatial orientation until much later, when the SMMSE score is in the low teens. Many of the fluctuations in Lewy body dementia look like delirium and it may, in fact, increase the predilection for delirium.

Patients with Lewy body dementia are exquisitely sensitive to certain medications so drugs should be introduced cautiously. Psychotrophic medications, particularly antipsychotics and anti-Parkinsonian drugs, may exacerbate confusion and psychosis. Clinically, Lewy body patients tolerate and respond well to anticholinesterases, which may improve cognition and significantly reduce hallucinations and delusions.[13] While traditional antipsychotics (butyrophenones and phenothiazines) are absolutely contraindicated, if absolutely necessary atypical antipsychotics can be introduced cautiously and kept at low doses.

VASCULAR DEMENTIA[4]

First described by Emil Kraepelin in 1910 as "arteriosclerotic insanity," after earlier work by Alzheimer and Binswanger, Vascular Dementia is the second or third most common dementia and can be difficult to diagnose.

The term encompasses cognitive impairment secondary to a number of conditions that compromise cerebral arterial supply, including small vessel disease and multi-infarct dementia. This complex disease, with many clinical presentations, is more common in men.

Diagnosis is made from a classic history that may include the following features: sudden onset; step-wise progression; cardiovascular risk factors (hypertension, diabetes, smoking, hyperlipidaemia, etc.); transient ischaemic attacks; and/or history (or evidence) of previous stroke on clinical assessment. Patients with vascular dementia of small vessel disease type are more likely to have depression than their multi-infarct or AD counterparts.

Depending on the area involved in Vascular Dementia, the presentation of DBD varies. Apart from anxiety from awareness of deficits, patients with Vascular Dementia tend to preserve insight longer than those with AD. In our experience, agitation is more common in Vascular Dementia than AD while delusions and hallucinations are less common. This awareness can cause anxiety and depression. The characteristic features of Vascular Dementia are: focal deficits, gait problems, early incontinence and physical deficits that exacerbate disability.

PARKINSON'S DISEASE WITH DEMENTIA[1,5,12]

Dementia is common in Parkinson's disease. Occuring in about one quarter of patients; it appears to be associated with depression and older age of onset[12]. Common behavioural symptoms are hallucinations, delusions and apathy. Well-formed and often frightening, hallucinations are frequent and are often related to dopaminergic agents. As with Lewy body dementia, anti-psychotic medications need to be used with care as they can exacerbate extrapyramidal symptoms.

One area where a diagnostic dilemma exists is in differential diagnosis of patients who overlap between Parkinson's disease, Parkinsonism and dementia. Up to 30% of patients with AD have features of Parkinsonism, and a cardinal feature of Lewy body dementia is Parkinsonism. Parkinson's disease itself usually presents with emotional flattening, slower thinking and slower response times, facial masking, axial rigidity (difficulty getting out of a chair), cogwheel rigidity, pill-rolling tremor, lack of arm swing and a history of "slowing down."

The history of onset of deficits (i.e., their sequence and timing at the beginning) is crucial to differentiate between the different dementias. Whether Parkinsonism or cognitive impairment began first is central to the differential diagnosis. Although a clear history is often difficult to obtain and there are obvious overlaps clinically between these conditions, if motor symptoms precede cognitive features by 12 months, this is considered Parkinson's disease with dementia. If cognitive features precede motor symptoms, the diagnosis is more likely AD with Parkinson's, or Lewy body dementia.

FRONTOTEMPORAL DEMENTIA[1,6]

Frontotemporal dementia (FTD) usually presents with behavioural problems before there is clinical evidence of cognitive decline. While Alzheimer's disease is primarily a cognitive disorder with associated behavioural dysfunction, frontotemporal dementia may be considered as primarily a behavioural disorder with secondary cognitive impairment. DBD is more common in FTD than AD[6].

The main area of neuronal loss is in the frontal lobes, and behaviours are often incongruous, with a bizarre kind of behaviour that is puzzling to on-lookers and often recounted by witnesses with residual disbelief. As this type of dementia is more common in males, with an earlier age of onset, clinicians should have a higher index of suspicion when patients (particularly males) present before the seventh decade with behavioural symptoms.

Historically, frontotemporal dementia was called **Pick's disease**. Pick's disease has focal cortical inclusion bodies primarily in the frontal lobes, with progressive aphasia, apraxia and agnosia. Recently, different pathologies have been identified that cause frontal atrophy without Pick bodies. Pick's disease is now recognized as a subset of these patients.

Frontotemporal dementia usually presents with socially inappropriate behaviour, insensitivity and **abulia** (lack of initiative and inability to make decisions). The patients' constructional and calculating abilities are preserved and their short-term memory is intact.

Behavioural disorders have an insidious onset, with slow progressive loss of social tact and self-awareness and growing disinhibition, impulsivity, inflexibility and rigidity. The emergence of repetitive, stereotyped behaviours and inability to manage personal hygiene and grooming are also suggestive of frontotemporal dementia. Some of these patients develop obsessive-compulsive features, with rituals. Others have severe apathy and emotional blunting. When patients present with apathy, imaging or EEG may be used to distinguish between depression and dementia. If the EEG is normal, depression is more likely. If the EEG shows focal slowing, and/or the CT, MRI, or single positron emission computerized tomography (SPECT) results show atrophy of the frontal lobes, frontotemporal dementia is more likely.

DEPRESSION-RELATED DEMENTIA[8,9,10]

Depression, common in the elderly, is even more common in dementia, occurring in up to 28% of patients[9]. Depression may be a risk factor for dementia and can be the presenting symptom[10].

Contributing factors that support a diagnosis of depression include the following: previous history or family history of depression, recent death(s) of family and/or friends, chronic pain, or loss of mobility, independence, sight or hearing. Vegetative signs, when present, also support the diagnosis. These include loss of appetite, sleep disturbance and low energy. Family and friends may complain of a particular event that preceded the change in function, or be able to pinpoint the time when the memory difficulty began. While the onset of a "classic" dementia such as Alzheimer's disease is insidious, gradual and progressive, usually over years, depression commonly comes on over months, even weeks. When patients with depression are questioned, particularly with the SMMSE, they may answer, "I don't know," or, "Who cares?" Some even ignore the questions.

Some depressed patients present with a "negative" behaviour profile that includes apathy, loss of interest and **anhedonia** (the hallmark of depression— loss of interest in, and withdrawal from, all regular and pleasurable activities). Another distinct presentation has more "positive" symptoms, with signs of anxiety, panic attacks, insomnia and hypochondriasis, involving multiple, changing somatic complaints. When a patient continues to complain and is convinced that "there is something wrong" despite repeated, thorough investigation of symptoms that are negative, and fails to respond to regular medical treatment, consider depression.

When depression presents like dementia, with memory loss and cognitive impairment, this is called **pseudodementia**. Differentiating dementia from pseudodementia can be difficult. Diagnosing depression in patients with significant cognitive impairment is also difficult, because the patient is unable to articulate his or her inner feelings and emotions. It is essential to take a collateral history from the caregiver. Depression is a huge contributor to the burden on caregivers, and caregivers of patients with dementia are at increased risk of depression. Depression in the patient is often accompanied by depression in the caregiver. Both may require treatment simultaneously.

ALCOHOL-RELATED DEMENTIA

Dementia is a common consequence of chronic alcoholism. It results, in part, from nutritional deficiencies, especially thiamine deficiency. Another factor is the probable toxic effects of chronic alcohol consumption, causing cerebral damage and consequent atrophy. Prolonged thiamine deficiency causes Korsakoff's syndrome—impairment in short-term recall, disorientation, confabulation and behavioural dysfunction. Mammillary body atrophy may be visible on an MRI scan.

NEW-VARIANT CREUTZFELD-JACOB DISEASE

New-variant Creutzfeld-Jacob disease (CJD), an extremely rare prion-transmitted disease, has achieved publicity recently in Europe. The hallmark is early behavioural symptoms with florid psychosis. The disease progress rapidly and patients develop myoclonic jerks or a "startle reflex," in which they jump and jerk suddenly and involuntarily. This is predominantly a disease of younger adults.

NORMAL PRESSURE HYDROCEPHALUS

Normal pressure hydrocephalus (NPH), an uncommon disorder, presents with the following clinical triad: dementia, gait disorder and incontinence— a common cluster of symptoms in patients with dementia. Failure to diagnose early can result in progressive deficits. Early and appropriate shunting may preserve function in some cases.

DELIRIUM

Delirium is common. It is considered a medical emergency that needs to be properly assessed and treated. In cognitively intact individuals it is obvious, but in people with cognitive impairment it is more difficult to interpret sudden changes in cognition. The common causes of delirium are anticholinergic drugs, dehydration, infections, acute cardiovascular or cerebrovascular events, metabolic disorders, pain and a sudden alteration in the environment. Patients who already have cognitive impairment are at increased risk.

The diagnostic criteria for delirium are the following:

- Disturbed sleep-wake cycle, with an acute or subacute onset; psychomotor and EEG disturbances; fluctuation and alterations in the level of consciousness; and perceptual disturbance (illusions or hallucinations).
- Evidence that the disturbance is caused by a general condition, like dehydration, pain and sepsis; substance abuse (intoxication or withdrawal); or multiple aetiologies.

A more rapid, florid onset of symptoms and signs also suggests delirium, rather than dementia, along with a disturbance in the level of consciousness that is only present in the later stages of dementia. Attention is more impaired in delirium than it is in dementia. In delirium, there is a marked disorientation, with incoherent speech, whereas in dementia, disorientation only occurs years after the onset. Perceptual disorders with early misinterpretations, illusions and hallucinations are common in delirium, and are not an early feature of dementia. Sleep/wake cycle is disturbed in delirium with swings of aggression, apathy and fearfulness. These are typically not early features of dementia. People with delirium are often frightened, hostile and/or fearful, while patients with dementia are more likely to be socially intact or anxious.

Lewy body dementia, and delirium, both have fluctuating deficits, visual hallucinations and delusions. Delirium is likely to have a more rapid onset with a more marked alteration in the level of consciousness than Lewy body disease. An absence of rigidity and Parkinsonism, with a reduced attention span and sleep/wake disruption, are also features of delirium rather than Lewy body disease. Delirium in Lewy body disease itself is well beyond the scope of this short book (and some could suggest, the authors' as well !)

CLINICAL GEMS

- The most common cause of dementia is Alzheimer's disease.
- Vascular dementia and Lewy body dementia account for the majority of the other cases.
- It is important to distinguish between the different dementias, depression and delirium, as this will have therapeutic and prognostic significance.
- Different dementias may co-exist, most commonly vascular and Alzheimer's disease, and this is called mixed dementia.
- DBD is common in each type of dementia and there are patterns of DBD that can be characteristic of each.
- Frontotemporal dementia has characteristic clustered features.
- Lewy body dementia and Parkinson's disease with dementia have similiar clinical features. Central to differentiation is the timing of onset of dementia and Parkinsonian features.
- Important differential diagnoses are depression and delirium. Differentiating between these two disorders presents a challenge to clinicians.

Table 4.1. Differential Diagnosis (with Common and Less Common Causes)

	ONSET	PROGRESSION	TYPICAL FEATURES	DIAGNOSIS	TREATMENT
ALZHEIMER DISEASE	Slow (years)	Gradual over years	• Normal attention • Short term memory loss • Disoriented to time • Repetitive • Unaware of, or conceals disabilities • Near-miss answers • Denial of problems • Head-turning sign	• Clinical: exclude other causes • CT/MRI: medial-temporal analysis	• Anticholinesterase • Vitamin E • Ginko • ASA • Multi-B vitamins • Modify cerebrovascular risk factors (e.g.,statins)
VASCULAR DEMENTIA	Abrupt (days)	Step-like	• History of stroke • Other atherosclerotic disease and risk factors • Focal neurological abnormalities e.g. gait and weakness • Depression often associated • Early incontinence • Apraxia/language spatial problems early • More anger and agitation less delusions than AD	• History • CT (brain) • MRI (superior) • Physical exam	• ECASA - Aspirin • Modify cerebrovascular risk factors
LEWY BODY DEMENTIA	Slow (years)	Fluctuating and progressive	• Fluctuating episodes of apparent confusion • Visual hallucinations • Extra-pyramidal features • Delusions • Gait abnormalities/falls • Walks "slumped over" • intolerant to neuroleptics	• History and physical exam	• Anticholinesterases • Avoid anti-psychotics if possible (use atypical) • Sodium valproate
PARKINSON'S DISEASE	Slow	Slow	• Pill-rolling tremor, bradykinesia, rigidity • Shuffling gait • Older age of onset of Parkinson's Disease	Clinical features and temporal relationship between motor and cognitive symptoms	• Anticholinesterases • Avoid anti-psychotics (atypical if necessary) • Adjust dopaminergic agents carefully

	ONSET	PROGRESSION	TYPICAL FEATURES	DIAGNOSIS	TREATMENT
FRONTO-TEMPORAL DEMENTIA	Slow (years)	Usually 2 to 7 years	• Early personality change • Euphoria • Emotional blunting • Obsessive features • Disinhibition • Apathy • Language difficulties • Explosive anger/agitation	SPECT/CT/MRI (frontal atrophy)	• SSRI • Atypical antipsychotic
NORMAL PRESSURE HYDRO-CEPHALUS	Slow	Variable	• Urinary incontinence • May have gait problem "glue-footed" (feet stuck to the floor) • Cognitive impairment • Gait or cognition may improve after removal of 40 to 50c.c. cerbrospinal fluid • Normal power and coordination in legs • May have history of trauma or meningitis	• Grossly dilated ventricles disproportionate to cortical atrophy	Refer to neurologist or neurosurgeon for opinion. Shunt may be of benefit.
PROGRESSIVE SUPRA NUCLEAR PALSY	Slow	Slow	• Vertical (supranuclear gaze paralysis • Startled /wide-eyed looking • Bradykinesia • Dysarthria (palatal speech) • Dysphagia (choking on food) • Gait disturbance (frequent falls) • No tremor • Extended neck posture • Poor response to levodopa	• History and examination	Symptomatic
PRIMARY PROGRESSIVE APHASIA	Slow	Slow	• At first, marked aphasia • Can maintain communication using non-speech methods • Maintain: - judgement - reasoning - memory - visuospatial skills • May progress to generalized dementia over time	• Aphasia with preserved cognition	Symptomatic

	ONSET	PROGRESSION	TYPICAL FEATURES	DIAGNOSIS	TREATMENT
CREUTZFELDT JAKOB DISEASE	Rapid	Very rapid progression (months)	• Younger patients, often with predominant psychotic symptoms • Muscle jerking, myoclonus • Person seems to be "shivering" - muscles twitch at rest • Mixed signs: pyramidal- extrapyramidal - cerebral • Characteristics EEG periodic 1-2 Hz pattern • Family history • Rare (20 cases/year in Canada)	Clinical features and EEG	Symptomatic
DEPRESSION	Rapid onset (weeks/-months)	Rapid	• Anhedonia • Depressed mood • "Don't know" answers • Diurnal variations (worse in a.m.) • Vegetative signs • History of depression • Disability gap • May have somatic delusions • Suicidal thoughts	Depression score	• Treat or remove cause • SSRI
DELIRIUM	Abrupt (days)	Rapid	• Acute illness • Attention deficit • Agitated/Frightened confused • Fluctuating level of consciousness • Sleep/waking disturbed hour to hour • Hallucinations/delusions	• Uncover cause, e.g., acute illness, drug, dehydration	Treat underlying cause
DEMENTIA PUGILISTICA	Slow	Slow	• "Fighter's" dementia • History of head injuries • Parkinson's symptoms : tremor, rigidity, unsteady gait • Memory loss progressive to dementia	History and clinical finding	May respond to levodopa

Chapter 5

ASSESSING AND MANAGING DBD

"Our mode of communication seems like under-
water sonar, each bouncing pulsations off the other,
and listening for an echo."
—*John Bailey, in "Iris: A Memoir of Iris
Murdoch."*

Learning objectives:
* Learn a user-friendly, quick guide to comprehensive assessment of dysfunctional behaviour in
  dementia (DBD).
* Learn to adapt standard approaches to history-
  taking and collateral history-taking. A reliable
  history is not always available from the patient

so it is important to get a history from the caregiver.

• Learn how to isolate and eliminate triggers of DBD.

• Learn to use the "ABCDE of Dementia" checklist for fast and thorough assessment.

• Gain practical tips on developing a care plan that has realistic goals.

• Gain the ability to evaluate treatment strategies. What works? What doesn't?

INTRODUCTION

The assessment of DBD is a critical part of the evaluation of any patient with dementia. The pattern and severity of DBD in people with cognitive impairment is determined by a number of factors, including the type of dementia, the severity of cognitive impairment and the internal and external environment. Appreciation and understanding of these concomitant features is crucial in the assessment and management of DBD.

Dysfunctional behaviour should be actively sought at each assessment to avoid a crisis later. Patients and caregivers both suffer the consequences of DBD and both require care. If clinicians wait until caregivers bring DBD to their attention, problems may not be addressed until they have reached a crisis point, and caregivers are burnt out.

At the assessment, the health care team needs to

take a comprehensive history, screen for DBD and develop a care plan to manage each behaviour that can be modified as the responses and needs of patients and/or caregivers change.

A detailed and comprehensive collateral history from the caregiver is critical because patients with DBD are often poor historians, have limited communication skills and frequently lack insight. Take the history from caregivers out of earshot of patients, otherwise caregivers may be reluctant to provide accurate accounts for fear of upsetting patients, who may not remember these episodes and will accuse caregivers of fabricating or exaggerating.

A useful approach to capturing a comprehensive assessment of DBD is to use the "ABCDE of Dementia" clinical tool (below), which offers a generic approach to each behaviour. Further examples of the use of the "ABCDE" are provided in Chapter 9.

THE "ABCDE DEMENTIA CHECKLIST"

The "ABCDE of Dementia" covers all the domains affected and places each behaviour in the context of the other domains. The five domains include:

"A"	- Activities of daily living (ADL) function
"B"	- Behaviour
"C"	- Cognition
"D"	- Depression
"E"	- Effects of the disease on the caregiver

Activities of Daily Living

ADL is measured quickly and reliably by asking the caregiver to fill out a simple instrument that measures independence in ADL (Clinical Tool 2, below). This provides a useful baseline and measure of function and disability.

Dysfunctional Behaviour

Frequency and impact of DBD is measured formally by asking caregivers to score a simple DBD assessment tool—the Dysfunctional Behaviour in Dementia Rating Instrument (DBDRI)[1] (Clinical Tool 3, below). This short screen provides a baseline to assess the effects of treatment over time.

Cognitive Function

Cognitive function is measured using the Standardized Mini Mental State Examination[2] (SMMSE) that takes about 10 minutes to complete.

Depression

The patient may be quickly screened for depression by asking the following for questions.[4,5] These will accurately **rule out** depression if they are negative (clear boxes).

	YES	NO
Are you basically satisfied with your life?		■
Do you feel happy most of the time?		■
Do you feel that your life is empty?	■	
Have you dropped many of your activities and interests?	■	

If one or more of these are positive, then inquire about vegetative signs:

	YES	NO
Do you feel full of energy?		■
Do you have trouble getting a good sleep?	■	
Do you think your mood is good?		■
Do you have a good appetite?		■
Do you think you'd be better off dead?	■	
Do you ever think about killing yourself?	■	

It is important to get a collaborative history from a family member or caregiver. If you suspect depression that has caused a change in function with a loss in quality of life, depending on the symptoms and vegetative signs, choose the most appropriate antidepressant. If one suspects the caregiver is also depressed, it is advisable to screen the caregiver as well.

Caregiver Burden

Caregiver burden may be assessed and scored using the Zarit burden scale[6] or some similar instrument.

Clinical Tool 1: The "ABCDE of Dementia Checklist"

The "ABCDE" is filled out as follows for a patient, Mr J., who presents with memory loss and disorientation:

ADL	Independent in basic ADL; however, gets lost driving and misses occasional stop signs, has problems paying bills and managing medications, and forgets appointments.
Behaviour	Frustrated, repeats questions and stories; lately has been getting angry with wife, shouting at her and accusing her of exaggerating his problems and making up stories.
Cognition	Scores 23/30 on the SMMSE; obvious difficulties in word finding and recall; disoriented to time; has impaired judgement because of lack of insight into deficits.
Depression	No insight, no mood change; energy, appetite and sleep unchanged.
Effects on Caregiver	Wife does not know how to handle his anger and accusations; she is afraid that he may get worse and does not know how to deal with the driving issues; he refuses to allow her to supervise his medications and pay bills; she has osteoporosis, is frail and anxious.

Clearly, in the case of Mr J., one would also review concomitant conditions and medications, and consider further investigations and treatments. Further examples of the use of the "ABCDE of Dementia" are provided in the case examples in Chapter 9.

The "ABCDE" is a simple checklist, that helps to frame clinical problems. When filled in comprehensively, it highlights the issues in each domain that need attention and ensures that no domain is forgotten or ignored. It prompts the physician to describe active issues and to develop simple strategies to address these problems.

Clinical Tool 2: Activities of Daily Living Score (ADLS)

THESE QUESTIONS ARE ABOUT HOW YOUR RELATIVE FUNCTIONS EVERY DAY.

WITH REGARD TO THE FOLLOWING FUNCTIONS, WHICH OF THESE STATEMENTS BEST DESCRIBES HOW YOUR RELATIVE HAS FUNCTIONED IN THE LAST WEEK?

Type of Activity of Daily Living	What is the Level of Care Required 1. Not applicable-never did this 2. Complete care required 3. Assistance required 4. Supervision required 5. Set-up required (physical) 6. Prompting required (verbal) 7. Performs spontaneously and independently	How Much of a Problem is this? 1. Great deal of problem 2. Quite a problem 3. Moderate problem 4. Somewhat of a problem 5. Little problem 6. Very little problem 7. No problem
Instrumental Activities of Daily Living (IADL)		
1. Transportation (car, taxi, or public transportation)	1 2 3 4 5 6 7	1 2 3 4 5 6 7
2. Finances (handling money, banking, bills)	1 2 3 4 5 6 7	1 2 3 4 5 6 7
3. Shopping (food, clothing, personal items)	1 2 3 4 5 6 7	1 2 3 4 5 6 7
4. Responsibility for medication (correct dosage and time)	1 2 3 4 5 6 7	1 2 3 4 5 6 7
5. Using the phone (dialing and answering)	1 2 3 4 5 6 7	1 2 3 4 5 6 7
6. Food Preparation (adequate meals and diet)	1 2 3 4 5 6 7	1 2 3 4 5 6 7
7. Housekeeping (adequate level of cleanliness)	1 2 3 4 5 6 7	1 2 3 4 5 6 7
8. Laundry (all personal and household)	1 2 3 4 5 6 7	1 2 3 4 5 6 7

IADL TOTAL _____

Type of Activity of Daily Living	What is the Level of Care Required	How Much of a Problem is this?
	1. Not applicable-never did this 2. Complete care required 3. Assistance required 4. Supervision required 5. Set-up required (physical) 6. Prompting required (verbal) 7. Performs spontaneously and independently	1. Great deal of problem 2. Quite a problem 3. Moderate problem 4. Somewhat of a problem 5. Little problem 6. Very little problem 7. No problem
Basic Activities of Daily Living (BADL)		
1. Walking	1 2 3 4 5 6 7	1 2 3 4 5 6 7
2. Tranfers (bed to chair)	1 2 3 4 5 6 7	1 2 3 4 5 6 7
3. Toileting (bladder and bowels)	1 2 3 4 5 6 7	1 2 3 4 5 6 7
4. Bathing (bath, shower, sponge bath)	1 2 3 4 5 6 7	1 2 3 4 5 6 7
5. Grooming (hair, nails, shaving, etc.)	1 2 3 4 5 6 7	1 2 3 4 5 6 7
6. Dressing (select clothes, dress/undress)	1 2 3 4 5 6 7	1 2 3 4 5 6 7
7. Feeding (eat food on plate/bowl)	1 2 3 4 5 6 7	1 2 3 4 5 6 7
BADL TOTAL	_____	_____
IADL and BADL TOTAL SCORE	_____	_____

Clinical Tool 3: Dysfunctional Behaviour in Dementia Rating Instrument (DBDRI)

HOW OFTEN HAS

....[

PATIENT'S NAME] HAD ANY OF THE FOLLOWING BEHAVIOURS IN THE LAST FEW WEEKS?

(Circle the number that best applies)

Type of Dysfunctional Behaviour	How Often Does This Occur? 0 Never / 1 About every two weeks / 2 About once a week / 3 More than once a week / 4 Atleast once daily / 5 More than five times a day						How Much of a Problem is this? 1 No problem / 2 Little problem / 3 Moderate problem / 4 Serious problem / 5 Very serious problem					
1.0 Dysfunctional Repetition												
1. Repeating questions or stories	0	1	2	3	4	5	0	1	2	3	4	5
2.0 Dysfunctional External Responses (Caregiver directed)												
1. Became angry	0	1	2	3	4	5	0	1	2	3	4	5
2. Was aggressive	0	1	2	3	4	5	0	1	2	3	4	5
3. Temper outbursts	0	1	2	3	4	5	0	1	2	3	4	5
4. Refused to co-operate	0	1	2	3	4	5	0	1	2	3	4	5
5. Demanding, calling out	0	1	2	3	4	5	0	1	2	3	4	5
6. Embarrassing behaviour in public	0	1	2	3	4	5	0	1	2	3	4	5

3.0 Dysfunctional Internal Responses (Patient distress)

1. Agitated	0	1	2	3	4	5
2. Crying	0	1	2	3	4	5
3. Frustrated	0	1	2	3	4	5

4.0 Dysfunctional Activities

1. Wandering	0	1	2	3	4	5
2. Up at night (sleep disturbance)	0	1	2	3	4	5
3. Afraid to be left alone	0	1	2	3	4	5
4. Became withdrawn	0	1	2	3	4	5
5. Wanted to leave	0	1	2	3	4	5

5.0 Dysfunctional Perceptions

1. Hallucinations	0	1	2	3	4	5
2. Delusions	0	1	2	3	4	5
3. Illusions	0	1	2	3	4	5
4. Hoarding/hiding	0	1	2	3	4	5

TOTAL _____

COMBINED TOTAL _____

WHAT TO DO WHEN DBD IS PRESENT

When dysfunctional behaviour is present in dementia, we recommend this practical five-step approach to assessment and management:
1. Describe the behaviour
2. Describe triggers and consequences
3. Develop realistic goals
4. Develop a care plan
5. Evaluate the treatment.

1. Describe the Behaviour

Describe and document the behaviour, its frequency and severity, and any associated risks. Describe the actual behaviour and don't make assumptions about any underlying causes. Describe what actually happens, for example, "he strikes out with his fist and shouts when I try to dress him," rather than, "he gets angry/ agitated/aggressive or resists care." The more detailed and specific the description of the actual behaviour, the better. Get the patient and caregiver to describe what happened and why.

Taking a history from the patient is usually of limited or of no value. Most behaviours are reported by caregivers and patients usually have limited insight, if they are, in fact, aware of the problems at all. This dependence on the caregiver for the history introduces informant bias: the caregiver's tolerance, emotional state, mood, coping ability and relationship with the patient affects the accuracy and validity of DBD reports. Health care professionals should be aware of this built-in bias in caregiver reports of dysfunctional behaviour; however, there is no foolproof way of getting absolutely accurate information unless one has the opportunity to speak to more than one observer—which is rare. Patients should not, however, be excluded from the discussion: their participation is useful to gather their perspectives, to try to make them more aware of the problems and to increase their compliance with treatment.

Along with a record of the frequency, duration and severity of DBD, you should attempt to determine whether patients or caregivers are at risk. For example, is the patient wandering and at risk of becoming lost, or could the caregiver be at risk of being injured by the patient?

2. Describe Triggers and Consequences

a) Define the Triggers

The four main triggers that exacerbate DBD are:
1. Caregiver behaviour

2. Level of patient's cognitive
   impairment

3. Current health status
   (e.g., pain, fecal impaction)

4. External environment.

These different factors do not exist in isolation but influence each other, so health professionals and caregivers need to understand their interplay and how they affect the clinical presentation of DBD. Caregivers should describe the triggers to health professionals so they can both learn to recognize possible triggers. For example, nocturnal wandering may be caused or exacerbated by pain, nocturia, paroxysmal nocturnal dyspnoea, early morning wakening, daytime napping, nightmares, misperceptions in the dark, caffeine at bedtime, noise and/or alterations in sleep patterns. In most cases in institutions, DBD is precipitated when others assist with ADL care such as bathing, dressing and changing.

Changes in current health status, such as respiratory tract infections, or changes in environment, such as crowded shopping centres, or tired, irritable caregivers, or frustration with word-finding may all trigger DBD. Management of the problem is based primarily on removing or mitigating these triggers.

b) Describe the Consequences of DBD

What happened when the patient displayed the behaviour? Did the caregiver become angry or frightened, try to reason with the person, or ignore the behaviour? Was this response helpful? Did it resolve the situation or did it promote more dysfunctional behaviour? Does the caregiver understand why the behaviour occurred, or does the caregiver think that the person is doing this to deliberately annoy him/her? Has the caregiver given up and decided to institutionalize the patient? How is this behaviour affecting the patient and caregiver? Is either of them depressed, anxious, or losing sleep? Has the DBD exacerbated other problems such as hypertension, dyspepsia, arthritis or angina?

c) Examine and Investigate

Physical examination identifies medical conditions that may cause or contribute to DBD. Investigations may include biochemical, serological, bacteriological or radiographic tests depending on the specific circumstances in each case.

3. Set Realistic Goals

DBD occurs in most patients with dementia and will persist in some cases for the rest of their lives. Goals of treatment should to be realistic. The physician, patient and caregiver need to be aware of what can be done. In many cases DBD cannot be eliminated completely but it can be improved. Many behaviours take time to respond to treatment. There is no magic bullet or instant cure, and medications should not be presented as such.

The failure to discuss, construct and present realistic goals will result in the caregiver becoming even more frustrated and angry and losing trust in the physician.

4. Develop a Care Plan

Once realistic goals have been developed, one needs to construct a plan of action. At this point the clinician should establish a process for implementing non-pharmacological and pharmacological interventions to treat the behaviour. Central to successful management is comprehensive assessment and accurate diagnosis. Management is directed at slowing deterioration and improving cognitive function. This is done by putting structures in place to reduce stress (where possible) and therapeutically manipulating chemicals in the brain.

Treatment will often take weeks rather than days to show effects. If medications are used, it is better to "start low and go slow" to minimize the risk of unwanted side effects that will lead to treatment failure. Starting at high doses actually loses time, rather than saving it.

5. Evaluate the Treatment

The effectiveness of the management plan can be clearly documented by repeating assessments such as the SMMSE, GDS, Zarit scale and/or DBDRI after treatment. The caregiver and the health care team should jointly decide on the intervals between assessments.

Clinical Tool 4: A Five-step Approach to DBD

1.	Describe the behaviour
2.	Describe triggers and consequences
3.	Set realistic goals
4.	Develop a careplan
5.	Evaluate treatment

CLINICAL GEMS

- Describe the behaviour objectively. Avoid making assumptions as to what emotion is displayed.
- If triggers are not recognized and eliminated, DBD will continue.
- Patients who have DBD usually continue to have it for the remainder of their lives. Realistic goals of management need to be developed, otherwise unrealistic expectations will fail and frustrate patients, caregivers and physicians, leading to more aggravation and premature institutionalization.
- DBD takes time to respond and it is better to start medications low and go slow. Starting higher will lead to more treatment failures from oversedation, akithesia and EPS (extra-pyramidal symptoms).
- Always review the effects of treatment.

Chapter 6

NON-PHARMACOLOGICAL MANAGEMENT

Learning Objectives:

- Become familiar with non-pharmacological interventions to manage dysfunctional behaviour in dementia (DBD).
- Gain familiarity with behavioural therapy for patients and caregivers.
- Be able to discuss coping strategies for caregivers.
- Understand the roles of psychotherapy, validation therapy, reminiscence therapy and reality orientation.

- Understand the role of the environment in prevention and treatment of DBD.
- Gain an appreciation of the importance of routines and maintaining daily activities.

THE IMPORTANCE OF PREVENTION

As in other areas in health care, it is important to emphasize prevention in the management of DBD. This is especially true of behavioural dysfunction because it's occurrence can have such devastating consequences for patients and caregivers. At each assessment, clinicians need to screen for DBD to diagnose early and start treatment as soon as possible before it escalates. Particular emphasis is directed at screening for depression because it is associated with more troublesome behavioural dysfunction.

Non-pharmacological treatment to modify the environment and remove triggers for dysfunctional behaviour is directed at both patients and caregivers. Clinical studies have clearly demonstrated the benefits to caregivers and patients of improved social support and education. [1,2,3] There is increasing interest in individualized patient approaches to therapy whereby patients' characteristics are taken into account when formulating each treatment approach.[4]

There are many ways of classifying non-pharmacological approaches; for example, emotional-orientated, stimulation-orientated, behaviour therapy and communication training.[5]

We have grouped them into five categories that may have more clinical applicability:

1. Behaviour modification approaches for the caregiver
2. Behaviour modification approaches for the patient
3. Environmental modification
4. Development and maintainence of routines
5. Sensory interventions.

BEHAVIOUR MODIFICATION FOR THE CAREGIVER

Our behaviour is influenced by those about us. Caregivers need to learn to prevent dysfunctional responses from patients by recognizing triggers and avoiding them. Behaviour is learned, and caregivers need to learn the most appropriate ways of approaching and responding to patients with cognitive impairment.

Learn Coping Strategies

- The health care team and caregivers should consider what has been successful in the past in preventing or reducing DBD when it occurred.
- Caregivers should keep a log of behaviours, triggers, actions taken and responses.
- Be calm and stand back whenever possible.
- Use calm voice, touch, music and familiar personal items to distract and promote tranquility

and relaxation.

• Reassure and comfort the patient.

Communicate

Reasoning is a common adult form of communication, but people with dementia have impaired reasoning from an early stage of the disease. Reasoning is likely to work only in the early stages, and in some cases may increase rather than decrease frustration levels. It is better to try to distract a patient who is angry or aggressive rather trying to reason with him/her to deal with the problem head on. Gentle touching, massage or hugging may be more effective than reasoning in soothing and comforting angry patients. Because people with dementia usually have language difficulties, gestures and actions can be more effective than verbal communication. Facial expression, posture, eye contact, tone of voice and gestures may be more effective than the actual words in relieving DBD.

People with dementia should be asked questions that can be answered simply, with yes/no answers. For example, rather than asking, "What flavour ice-cream would you like?," try, "Would you like ice-cream?" Caregivers should give the person enough time to respond, before proceeding with the next question, i.e., "Would you like strawberry ice cream?" They should be advised to present easy options and only give one at a time. They should also allow adequate time for the patient to process the information. Finding the right words can be difficult, so if the patient becomes frustrated, the caregiver should change the subject or create a diversion.

Those who care for people with dementia need to appreciate that people with dementia are not responsible, do not act intentionally, and cannot control their urges and dysfunctional behaviours. Patients should not be punished because they will not learn from criticism or negative reinforcement, which is likely to just make behaviour even worse.

At diagnosis, the caregiver should be referred to the local branch of the Alzheimer's society for education about the disease and access to the supports provided.

BEHAVIOUR MODIFICATION FOR THE PATIENT

Psychotherapy[6]

This type of therapy is usually carried out by psychologists and is generally reserved for patients with mild cognitive impairment. Its goal is to improve self-image and social interactions by improving communication skills and limiting socially dysfunctional behaviours. This form of therapy has its advocates but its widespread use is limited by the large amount of time it requires. It may be useful in some patients with very mild cognitive impairment and depression. Certain caregivers are more likely to benefit from psychotherapy and this is an important option in managing DBD and in supporting and maintaining caregivers.

Validation Therapy[5]

Developed in the 1980s, validation therapy focuses on the underlying emotional tone and context rather than what is actually being said by the patient. Therapy is geared at responding to the emotion rather than trying to respond to the content by reasoning with the person. This approach works well for people who have dementia as it permits communication in those with significant cognitive impairment. Caregivers respond to patients' emotional needs and thus avoid frustrating them if they fail to articulate their specific needs.

Reminiscence Therapy

Patients are encouraged to recount experiences that have occurred in the past without paying particular attention to details. This enables them to learn coping strategies from previous experiences and maintain their sense of identity. This technique also helps caregivers, as it allows improved insight into the condition by highlighting the discrepancy between long- and short-term memory. Nursing home residents may particularly benefit from this therapy.

Therapeutic Activities[7]

Therapeutic activities include creative arts

therapy. This form of therapy plays to patients' strengths and avoids the presumption that dementia removes a person's ability to be productive or creative. Time is taken to ascertain each person's interests and strengths so activities can focus on their favourite creative expression e.g., dance, art, music and/or literature.

Reality Orientation[8]

This type of therapy is used in patients who have mild cognitive impairment and disorientation. There are two forms: **24-hour** and **classroom**. The 24-hour technique involves staff verbally re-orientating the patient at every opportunity. In the classroom mode, 30-minute intensive re-orientation is given each day. Popular in the 1960s and 70s, reality orientation is used infrequently now, mainly because it can increase patients' awareness of their losses, promote frustration, and even worsen symptoms of anxiety and depression in people with moderate or severe dementia. We would not recommend it routinely.

MODIFICATION OF THE ENVIRONMENT

Adapt the Environment

People with dementia should be able to move about and exercise as they wish. Extremes of temperatures should be avoided and patients should wear sensible clothing, avoiding clothes with complicated zippers or buttons.

Caregivers should review the contents of the home and remove hazardous objects such as power tools, guns, sharp knives and dangerous appliances. Surprises should be avoided as much as possible, as changes to daily routine can increase frustration, disorientation, stress and irritability. People with dementia often cannot tolerate crowds or deal with more than a few people at a time. Multiple stimuli can increase stress, frustration, confusion and disorientation.

Milieu Therapy[9]

The environment with which patients interact, including the people in it, is referred as the therapeutic milieu. The therapeutic milieu has an essential bearing on all behaviour, but especially on "response" or "reaction" behaviours. Milieu therapy aims to manipulate the environment to encourage healthy interactions with the surroundings and the people who occupy it. Creativity and flexibility are two central qualities of a healthy or appropriate environment. Each environment is, where possible, individualized to the specific needs of each individual. For example, when elderly adults with dementia are transferred to a nursing home, it is important to furnish their room with familiar objects like photographs of family, furniture from home and flowers picked from their garden.

Institutional Environment

All institutional environments should be restraint free. Institutions with low restraint use have a higher proportion of residents active during the day. The units tend to be smaller in size, there are lower levels of functional dependence and fewer co-morbid conditions, with a lower prevalence of DBD[10]. The prevalence of DBD in institutions is dependent on the manner in which staff members treat patients and the physical design of the buildings where they live. The **Eden Alternative**, the development of a home-like environment in the nursing home, is one example of environmental and behavioural change on the part of staff and families that can improve quality of life and DBD in institutions.[17]

Behavioural Intensive Care Units (BICUs)[11]

Despite the premise that patients with DBD should be nursed in environments that are familiar and responsive to their needs, on some occasions DBD cannot be managed in the home. Aggressive behaviour is the most problematic behaviour for caregivers. In these cases, the ideal setting is an environment where specially trained staff are equipped to meet patients' needs—the behavioural intensive care unit.

Initially, the emphasis is on treating the behaviour and removing underlying triggers. Ideally, this is done using a multidisciplinary approach involving physicians, psychiatrists, trained nursing staff and allied health care professionals. Unfortunately, the majority of patients admitted to behavioural intensive care units subsequently require long-term care. This is not a result of poor care, but rather reflects the severity of DBD that led to admission.

Overall, BICUs can successfully reduce DBD, most commonly agitation and aggression (30% symptom reduction in 70% of patients) and are better alternatives than the more common practice of admitting people to acute medical wards, where staffing levels and training are often inadequate.

DEVELOP AND MAINTAIN ROUTINES

Routines provide people with dementia with a regular, reassuring framework within which to function. It is useful to create and maintain a routine by doing the following:
- Having meals at the same time every day.
- Scheduling activities like walking, shopping, music, cooking, cleaning, family visits and bedtime, at the same time each day as much as possible.
- Involving patients in these regular activities as much as possible.
- Allowing adequate time so patients are not rushed.
- Reconsidering activities that require adaptation to new circumstances, e.g., out-of-town trips.

Organize Activities

Caregivers and patients may withdraw from social activities due to embarrassment, disinterest and/or reduced mobility. However, people with dementing illnesses are more likely to develop behavioural symptoms if they stop their daily activities and routines. Regular physical activity is important and should be adapted according to each patient's fitness, likes and preferences. Some people enjoy group activities, others don't. Organized daily walks are particularly effective in reducing wandering, aggression and agitation. Activity should be invigorating, and not frustrating or tiring.

If the patient is having a bad day it may be advisable to cancel activities that day. If it is clear that an activity is going to cause problems, avoid it. For example, if the patient does not want to shower, leave it for the next day or try again later.

5. SENSORY INTERVENTIONS

Massage and Touch Therapy[13]

Touch is considered a therapeutic intervention by many nursing home staff. Dementia sufferers experience social isolation, lack of personal contact and are very responsive to this "hands-on" approach. Touch has a comforting and calming effect and is often used by caregivers because it has a beneficial effect on agitation, wandering, sleep/wake disruption and anxiety.

Bright Light Therapy[14]

This type of therapy may reinforce circadian rhythms and has been successfully used to treat sleep/wake disturbances.

Music Therapy[15,16]

Relaxing, "classical" music has been clinically demonstrated to reduce agitated behaviours. This is not surprising, given that music has an impact on the emotions. When using music as an intervention, it is important to use familiar music that suits the person's taste.

Music therapy is an under-rated and under-utilized intervention for agitated and aggressive behaviour. If it were available in pill form it might be prescribed and used more by physicians!

Pet Therapy[18]

The introduction of pet dogs has been shown to reduce agitation (especially sundowning), increase socialization and have an overall calming effect on patients with dementia.

CLINICAL GEMS

- Non-pharmacological approaches to treatment are often common sense measures.
- Non-pharmacological approaches are commonly underutilized but are effective intervention in the treatment of DBD.
- Non-pharmacological treatment should be considered first-line therapy, with drug therapy as an adjuvant.
- They can be used for acute therapy, but also for primary and secondary prevention of DBD.
- Caregivers should aim to create both internal and external environments from the earliest stages of dementia that prevent DBD.

Chapter 7

PHARMACOLOGICAL TREATMENTS

"Above all else, do no harm."

—Hippocrates

Learning Objectives:
- Become familiar with all medications that are used to treat dysfunctional behaviour in dementia (DBD).
- Understand the importance of drug dosages in relation to efficacy, but more importantly, side-effect profile.
- Learn patience: understand the relationship between commencing therapy and time to respond.

- Gain an understanding of where each of these medications is indicated.
- Become familiar with recent advances in antipsychotic medications, i.e., atypical antipsychotics, and how clinical practice has changed as a result of these new medications.

ANTIPSYCHOTICS [1,2]

- Most Antipsychotics exert their main effects on dopamine receptors in the mesolimbic, striatal and mesocortical systems. They have a consistent and reliable therapeutic effect in the treatment of many types of DBD. They are mainly used for dysfunctional responses (aggression, agitation) and dysfunctional perceptions (delusions and hallucinations) .
- "Traditional" antipsychotics are effective in DBD, but have significant toxicity and side effects (see below). Their detrimental effects are exacerbated in older adults by the longer duration of these drugs in the body, due to the greater volume of distribution and slower metabolism of antipsychotics in these patients. Older adults are also more sensitive to the toxic effects of antipsychotics.

Despite their unacceptable side-effect profiles, traditional antipsychotics are still indicated to control acute, severe agitation or aggression. They should be used for a short period i.e. <48hrs and are no longer recommended as drugs of first choice in the chronic management of DBD.

The recent development of "atypical" antipsychotics has made antipsychotics safer and more accessible to older adults. Atypical antipsychotics have comparable efficacy but dramatically better side-effect profiles than traditional antipsychotics.

Traditional Antipsychotics

Historically, these were the most widely used medications in the treatment of DBD and have only recently been overtaken by the atypical antipsychotics. They are more commonly used in men than women, probably because men are more likely to exhibit behavioural problems such as aggression, wandering, agitation and dangerous or socially inappropriate behaviours.

In general, about 60% of people with Alzheimer's disease (AD) who have psychotic symptoms with delusions, hallucinations, paranoia and/or aggression, respond modestly to antipsychotics.[3]

Traditional antipsychotics worsen the negative features of dementia such as cognitive impairment, apathy, withdrawal, amotivation and akinesia. Long-term use of traditional antipsychotics in older adults increases the risk of inducing extra-pyramidal effects (EPEs) and tardive dyskinesia.

Traditional antipsychotics are broadly divided into two main classes: the **phenothiazines** and the **butyrophenones**.

Phenothiazines

The phenothiazines (chlorpromazine, thioridizine, trifluoperazine and acetophenazine) were first developed in the 1950s. They revolutionized the treatment of psychotic conditions and helped to end life-long institutionalization of the psychotic, mentally ill. They are commonly used in DBD, and chlorpromazine is the most widely used drug in this class.

Overall, while response rates vary in different studies, phenothiazines have an efficacy rate of 59% for thioridizine[3] and 64% for acetophenzine[4].

The side effects of these medications include sedation, postural hypotension, dry mouth, blurred vision and constipation. Their sedative properties may be of benefit in some clinical situations where insomnia is a problem.

Butyrophenones

Butyrophenones e.g. haloperidol, were the most widely used antipsychotics until the late 1990s, when haloperidol was overtaken by the atypical antipsychotic, risperidone.

The butyrophenones reduced DBD (mainly symptoms of agitation and aggression) by about 60% in randomized, controlled trials.[5,9] Their main drawbacks are EPEs, pseudo-Parkinson's syndrome, tardive dyskinesia and akithesia (restless legs), as a result of dopamine blockade. As many as 50% of elderly patients treated with butyrophenones develop EPEs. In this group of patients, the risk of developing tardive dyskinesia with haloperidol is 28% after 1 year, 50% after 2 years and 63% after 3 years, even on low doses.[6]

For these reasons, this class of drugs should be avoided, particularly in those who already have extra-pyramidal symptoms and signs, i.e., patients with Lewy body dementia and Parkinson's disease with dementia.

Atypical Antipsychotics

Clearly, the traditional antipsychotics were less than satisfactory and the need for treatments with more favourable side-effect profiles was evident. The atypical antipsychotics were developed to meet this need. Four atypical antipsychotics are currently available: risperidone, olanzapine, clozapine and quetiapine.

Studies show that atypical antipsychotics are almost as effective as the traditional antipsychotics in managing the positive features of DBD (e.g., aggression, agitation), but they have clear advantages in their effect on the negative features (e.g., impairments in cognition and the ability to perform activities of daily living (ADL).

Risperidone and olanzapine, for example, cause much less impairment of cognition than traditional antipsychotics, and fewer EPEs at efficacious doses. In one study, EPEs occurred in 7% on risperidone, 22% on haloperidol and 18% on thioridizine.[8] When loxapine, a medium-potency agent, and haloperidol were compared, loxapine was shown to have comparable efficacy with fewer side effects. [9]

Atypical antipsychotics will produce EPEs at higher doses, therefore one **must choose the right drug at the right dose.**

Due to their comparatively recent entry into the field, there is less clinical data available on atypical antipsychotics than the traditional antipsychotics in the treatment of DBD; the majority of the data is on risperidone. In many countries, risperidone is the most widely used antipsychotic for DBD.

Risperidone

Between 0.25 and 2.0 mg/day of risperidone is given in single or divided doses.

There are two published randomized, controlled trials with risperidone in the elderly with dementia, one compared it to placebo and another compared it to haloperidol.

In the first study, Katz et al. [10] studied the efficacy of risperidone in a double-blind, placebo-controlled trial involving 625 nursing home patients. In this cohort, 73% of patients had AD, 15% had vascular dementia and 12% had mixed dementias. The sample included severely demented people with a mean Mini Mental State Examination (MMSE) score of 6.6 at baseline. Four groups were randomized to either placebo, or 0.5 mg, 1.0 mg or 2.0 mg of risperidone daily for 12 weeks. The outcome was assessed using the Behavioural Pathology in Alzheimer's Disease Rating Scale (BEHAVE AD)[30].

The study showed that risperidone at doses of 1.0 mg and 2.0 mg daily was significantly more effective in reducing DBD than placebo, and it was not associated with significant deficits in cognition or self-care. Total rates of treatment discontinuation from adverse events were similar in patients who received placebo and risperidone, in doses of risperidone up to 1.0 mg daily.

A second double-blind, randomized, controlled trial compared risperidone with haloperidol in institutionalized older adults with DBD[11]. There were 344 patients admitted to the study, and each patient was randomized to receive either placebo, risperidone (0.5 mg to 4.0 mg daily) or haloperidol. The mean doses used were 1.2 mg of haloperidol and 1.1 mg of risperidone. Patients were followed for 12 weeks and the primary outcome was the percentage of patients with a 30% or greater improvement from baseline to endpoint on the BEHAVE AD total score. Patients were equivalent at baseline, with a mean MMSE score of about 8, with aggressiveness as the dominant behavioural feature.

Results demonstrated that in the risperidone, haloperidol and placebo groups, 72%, 69% and 61% respectively had at least a 30% reduction in BEHAVE AD scores at week 12. Risperidone had a significantly greater reduction in severity and frequency of behavioural symptoms than placebo. Risperidone was especially effective with aggressive behaviour at week 12, and there was significantly more improvement with risperidone than haloperidol on the BEHAVE AD aggressiveness score.

When it came to adverse events, the effects of risperidone were independent of sedation, and the number of patients who experienced EPEs on risperidone was not significantly different from that of placebo. By contrast, patients experienced more severe EPEs on haloperidol than placebo. There was no significant decline in cognitive function with risperidone (MMSE -0.5), but a significant deterioration was seen in cognitive function in the haloperidol group (MMSE -2.1) compared to placebo (MMSE +0.5). There was no difference in global dementia rating scales between the three groups. Total adverse event rates were 76.5%, 80% and 72.8% for risperidone, haloperidol and placebo respectively. Overall, there was no significant difference in the incidence of serious or adverse events between groups.

These two trials showed that risperidone controlled DBD, particularly aggressive behaviour without sedation, and without any significant increase in EPEs or reductions in cognition. Haloperidol, on the other hand, effectively treated the DBD but there was with a significant increase in EPEs and a significant reduction in cognition. Based on this evidence, we can conclude that risperidone is not a chemical restraint but a psychotherapeutic agent. These differences in frequency of EPEs and cognitive effects between risperidol and haloperidol are clinically significant and give risperidol a clear clinical advantage. Although these two studies were conducted on severely demented, institutionalized older adults with DBD, these differences may be even more important in community- living patients with DBD, where the development of EPEs and negative effects on cognition could increase disability and hasten institutionalization.

Olanzapine

A recent RCT[13] has demonstrated Olanzapine to be an effective treatment for DBD. A multicenter, double-blind, placebo-controlled 6 week study was conducted in 206 elderly US nursing home residents with AD and psychotic and/or agitation/aggression. At doses of 5 and 10mg, Olanzapine was significantly superior to placebo in treating agitation, aggression and psychotic symptoms without significantly affecting cognition or causing extrapyramidal side-effects relative to placebo. Patients receiving 5mg/day improved more than patients receiving 10mg/day. Patients receiving 15mg/day were no better than placebo. In this study, best results were achieved at lower doses ie., 5mg/day. The benefit in reducing DBD appeared to be lost when the dosage was increased to 15mg demonstrating the importance of correct dosaging. Comparative studies between risperidone and olanzapine do not exist in this group. However, a study[37] comparing olanzapine and risperidone in patients with Schizophrenia demonstrated an advantage with olanzapine in the effect on negative symptoms.

However, doses used in this study were much higher than those recommended in the elderly.

Olanzapine is given in single or twice-daily doses of 2.5 mg HS and is increased by increments of 2.5 mg, up to a maximum of 5.0 to 7.5 mg daily, the optimal dose in frail, older adults.

Quetiapine

Studies are underway, but there are currently no results available from double-blind, randomized trials of quetiapine in older adults with DBD.

A single study published on quetiapine's use in elderly patients with psychotic disorders demonstrated it to be effective and well tolerated.[12]

The two antipsychotic's that do not have D2 antagonist effects are clozapine and quetiapine. They do not cause any EPS and will not worsen symptoms of Parkinson's Disease. Quetiapine does not have the hematological side effects associated with clozapine. Quetiapine is now widely used in Parkinson's Disease and Lewy Body Dementia. Quetiapine is usually given once a day, staring with 12.5 to 25mg at bedtime. The dose is increased depending on the patients' tolerance and response. Most cases respond to 100mg/day taken at bedtime.

Clozapine

Clozapine is not used often but in some severely refractory cases it may be very useful. Clozapine was the first available atypical antipsychotic. Its use has been limited by a increased risk of agranulocytosis which is more marked in the elderly. [31] If used, blood counts must be monitored regularly.

Clozapine is generally used in the following circumstances:

• When target symptoms such as aggressive behaviour due to psychosis have not responded to traditional or novel antipsychotics
• If there is tardive dyskinesia limiting the use of traditional or other novel antipsychotics
• If patients with Parkinson's disease are unable to tolerate other antipsychotics[32].

The advantage of clozapine is that it does not cause extrapyramidal symptoms or tardive dyskinesia.

However, clozapine may cause agranulocytosis (which is reversible if the drug is stopped). The agranulocytosis is not dose-dependent and is, apparently, idiosyncratic; if agranulocytosis occurs the drug must be stopped, not reduced.

Because of this, when clozapine is used the patient must be monitored by weekly white cell counts for the first 26 weeks and every 2 weeks thereafter for the entire length of time that the patient is on the drug.

The starting dose of the clozapine in the elderly is 6.25 mg at night. The dose is then increased in increments of 6.25 mg according to tolerance and efficacy. Target dose is around 25 to 50 mg for Parkinson's psychosis, and in some cases may go to 300 mg. Aggressive symptoms will respond within a week or two. Full response will occur in 12 weeks.

Patients who are taking clozapine must be registered in the Clozaril® Support and Assistance Program, administered by the drug's manufacturer, Novartis. Phone 1-800-267-2726 for further information if you are thinking of prescribing clozapine.

Antipsychotics: Conclusions

There has been much debate about the choice between atypical and traditional antipsychotics. For the clinician and caregiver, the potential to avoid the debilitating side effects of traditional antipsychotics in frail, unsteady and confused older adults may make the choice of atypical antipsychotics easier. The advantages of atypical antipsychotics may be even more significant in a community setting, although further studies are needed. On balance we use and recommend atypical antipsychotics, because they do less harm.

Quetiapine appears promising and is widely used, particularly in patients with Parkinson's Disease or Lewy Body Dementia, although published, randomized, controlled trials and/or comparative data in the elderly with cognitive impairment is lacking. There is growing evidence to support the use of Olanzapine as effective therapy. In the absence of further evidence, risperidone is currently recommended as the first-line atypical antipsychotic in sub-acute and chronic treatment of aggression, agitation and psychosis in older patients with dementia because it has the strongest evidence to support its use. Treatment should be individualized. For example, if delusions or aggression are worse at night olanzapine may be indicated because of its sedative properties. Otherwise, risperidone would be indicated.

Table 7.1. Comparison between side effects of conventional and atypical antipsychotics

SIDE EFFECT	CONVENTIONAL ANTIPSYCHOTICS	ATYPICAL ANTIPSYCHOTICS			
		Clozapine	Risperidone	Olanzapine	Quetiapine
EPS	+/+++	0	0/+	0/+	0
TD	+/+++	0/+	0/+	0/+	0/+
Seizures	0/+	+++	0	0	0
Sedation	+/+++	+++	+	++	++
Anticholinergic	+/+++	+++	0	+	0
Orthostatic Hypotension	+/+++	+++	0/+	0/+	++
Weight Gain	+	+++	0/+	+++	++

ANTIDEPRESSANTS [17]

Antidepressants are effective and well tolerated in patients with depression and AD. SSRIs should theoretically be effective in Alzheimer's disease and DBD because of a demonstrated association between serotonergic dysfunction and aggressive behaviour in animal models. However, convincing evidence from clinical trials is lacking. Citalopram was used in one multi-centered trial[16] of patients with dementia, and reduced disruptive vocalizations, confusion, and restlessness. A small study examined the use of SSRIs in the treatment of DBD in frontotemporal dementia.[15] Despite the small numbers in the study, SSRIs improved symptoms in about 50% of patients.

In clinical practice, antidepressants are often used empirically, either alone or in combination with antipsychotics. We recommend their adjuvant, empirical use in patients with aggressive behaviour because of the high clinical correlation between depression and aggression.

Trazadone, a serotonergic antidepressant with alpha2-adrenergic blocking activity is frequently used in patients with DBD. One double-blind, randomized study[14] of trazadone in DBD patients demonstrated a 71% reduction in agitation and aggression, with a more favourable side-effect profile than haloperidol. It appears to be particularly effective for verbal aggression and repetitive behaviours. Trazadone is also of benefit in situations where nocturnal sedation is desired, when it is started at 25 to 50 mg at night. It is a frequently used as an adjuvant therapy to antipsychotics in agitated patients, especially if agitation is worse at night.

ANXIOLYTICS [18]

Benzodiazepines (BZD) are widely used in the acute treatment of DBD, primarily agitation and aggression, especially when there is an associated sleep disturbance. Generally, there is lack of consistency in comparative studies with antipsychotics in this population. Patients with dementia taking BZDs occasionally become more disinhibited and this can result in increased agitation. More severely demented and agitated patients are not helped by BZDs. There is also concern that they cause sedation, which can increase confusion and instability, and the risk of falls.

Short-acting benzodiazepines like lorazepam are useful in managing acute episodes of agitation and / or aggression, with the aim of preventing patients from injuring themselves or others. They are usually given with antipsychotics, or alone, as clinically indicated. They can also be used as short-term sedatives for special procedures such as CT scans. Alprazolam has been shown to be as effective as low-dose haloperidol in DBD.[19] Short-acting benzodiazepines have also been used in patients with Alzheimer's disease and disabling myoclonus.

BETA-BLOCKERS

Reports[34, 35] suggest that beta-blockers are effective in treating the symptoms of DBD particularly aggression and impulsivity, but there are no randomized, controlled trials in elderly demented patients. The main limitation to their use is concern about their side-effect profile in the elderly, which includes bradycardia (therefore should be used cautiously with anti-cholinesterases), hypotension, lethargy and bronchospasm. Propranolol and Pindolol are the most commonly used.

ANTICONVULSANTS

Anticonvulsants are an effective and promising treatment in DBD, where they can be used for agitation, aggression and emotional lability. Carbamazepine and valproic acid are most commonly used.[20]

Carbamazepine has psychotropic properties and is less neurotoxic than lithium, at least in the treatment of bipolar disorders. Three randomized, controlled trials reported the use of carbamazepine in DBD. In two studies where 300 mg/day were used, 64 to 77% of patients had a reduction in DBD (agitation and aggression), with an associated reduction in staff time needed to manage the DBD. The study that used lower doses of carbamazepine reported no response compared to placebo. Use of carbamazepine is limited by side effects and the absence of published multicentred trials.[21,22]

Valproic acid enhances gamma-aminobutyric acid (GABA)-mediated neurotransmission and has a more favourable side-effect and drug interaction profile than carbamazepine. However, it has been less well researched. While no randomized, controlled trials have examined the efficacy of valproic acid, there have been several open-label studies that suggest modest improvement in DBD at doses ranging from 750 to 2250 mg/day. [23,24,25]

Guidelines on the use of the anticonvulsants favour the use of valproic acid over carbamazepine because of valproic acid's more favourable side-effect and drug interaction profile. No studies have yet reported using the newer anticonvulsants such as Gabapentin in DBD.

MAO INHIBITORS[26]

The primary indication for selegiline, an irreversible monoamine oxidase type B inhibitor, is the treatment of Parkinson's disease. Several studies have shown improvements in behavioural scores in DBD with this medication but to date there have been no randomized, controlled trials confirming its efficacy.

HORMONE THERAPY[33]

A few case reports suggest that hormone therapy may be helpful for physical aggression associated with inappropriate sexual behaviour in men. Anti-androgen therapy reduces aggression, pacing, dysfunctional sexual behaviour and agitation in men. The dose for oral conjugated estrogens ranges from 0.625 to 1.25 mg/day and for medroxyprogesterone IM, 25 to 75 mg/week. GnRH analogues like leuprolide have also been used with some success but numbers in the trials were small. The side effects of anti-androgens in men are significant and current evidence does not support their use as a first-line treatment. Hormone therapy should be viewed as third-line treatment of aggressive behaviour in males.

BUSPIRONE

Buspirone is a partial 5-HT 1A agonist. There is no clear evidence to support its routine use in DBD. A comparative study[27] between trazadone and buspirone failed to demonstrate a statistically significant reduction in DBD. However, other studies have demonstrated a benefit with buspirone on symptoms of agitation[36].

CHOLINESTERASE INHIBITORS[28,29]

Cholinesterase inhibitors (anticholinesterases) have psychotropic activity, and beneficial effects on a wide range of behaviours, especially apathy, hallucinations, delusions, agitation and disinhibition. This effect can be attributed in part to the positive effects of cholinesterase inhibitors on cognition. The beneficial effect of these drugs may have a neurobiological basis that is mediated through limbic cholinergic structures. Anticholinesterases have been shown to reduce hallucinations and delusions in patients with Lewy body disease[38].

We recommend commencing donepezil at 5 mg daily and increasing to 10 mg after one month or Galantamine 4mg twice daily or Rivastigmine 1.5 mg twice daily to start.

CHLORAL HYDRATE

Chloral hydrate, first developed in 1869, the first synthetic hypnotic is one of the oldest sedatives, and. A solid, it is usually given orally in liquid form because it is so irritating to the stomach. Chloral hydrate tastes horrible so it is usually given with milk or juice. It induces sleep in about half an hour and its effects last for about 6 to 8 hours. It is rapidly metabolized by alcohol dehydrogenase and leaves very little or no hangover. Given with food, it can also be used for daytime behavioural problems, e.g., aggression or lability, in lower doses. The hypnotic dose is 0.5 to 2.0 grams, or for daytime behavioural problems, it is given as 0.25 to 0.5 grams up to three times a day, provided it does not produce sedation.

The main advantages of chloral hydrate are the low cost and the slight chance of build-up, or toxicity in the form of extrapyramidal syndrome or anticholinergic effects.

111

CLINICAL GEMS

- Medications are adjuvant therapy to non-pharmacological measures.
- Do not expect a "quick fix" with medications. Start low and go slow.
- Avoid using traditional antipsychotics except in the acute setting where parenteral therapy is required.
- Choice of medications should be individualized in a risk versus benefit approach.
- Have a high clinical suspicion for depression in patients with aggression.

Chapter 8

MANAGING SPECIFIC BEHAVIOURS

Learning Objectives:

- Become familiar with a systematic approach to categorizing dysfunctional behaviour in dementia (DBD).
- Gain a multi-faceted (pharmacological and non-pharmacological) approach to managing acute and chronic DBD.
- Develop a full understanding of the inter-relationship between the different types of dysfunctional behaviours.

- Understand how different behaviours manifest in different types of dementia.

In this chapter we describe the assessment and management of some specific behaviours, with examples from each of the four DBD categories described in Chapter 3. Most of the common behaviours are discussed, along with practical strategies for dealing with them. Chapter 9 gives cases with examples of these strategies in practice.

DYSFUNCTIONAL REPETITIONS

Repetitive Behaviours

Repetitive behaviours, common presenting symptoms in both Alzheimer's disease (AD) and frontotemporal dementia, may take the form of repeating sentences, questions, movements or gestures. Patients with premorbid obsessive-compulsive traits or neuroses are at increased risk of this type of DBD.

In frontotemporal dementia [1], the most common repetitive behaviour at presentation is repeatedly checking doors, windows, and so on.

Treatment for repetitive behaviour is only initiated when necessary and the decision to initiate treatment is usually at the caregiver's request, as this behaviour often does not cause patients any significant problems. Caregivers should start with simple behavioural measures, and remember that each time the patients ask questions, they think it is their first time. When the same question is repeated over and over, and the patient is in the early stages of dementia with relatively well preserved cognition, it is often helpful to have written answers to the question left about the house. If a particular object precipitates questions (e.g., the telephone), then the answer may be left next to the object. This simple measure is often effective.

In one small study, playing classical and favourite music to institutionalized patients with disruptive, repetitive vocalization reduced the disruptive pattern[2]. Clomipramine may be helpful[3], but further research is needed before it can be recommended for routine use in repetitive behaviour. Despite the absence of evidence, SSRI's appear to be a logical treatment option and are often tried in clinical practice.

Repetitive behaviour can change with different degrees of cognitive impairment. It is often difficult to distinguish between vocally disruptive and repetitive behaviour in severely demented nursing home residents.

DYSFUNCTIONAL RESPONSES

Aggression (See Case 5, Chapter 9)
Aggression may be physical (kicking, shoving, punching) or non-physical (name calling, shouting obscenities). Many patients with dementia exhibit aggressive symptoms at some stage in their illness.

Aggression is associated with a poorer prognosis and is a strong predictor of institutionalization[19]. It can be hazardous not only for caregivers but also for patients, who are often treated more like criminals (for example, by being jailed with physical restraints and antipsychotics) than people who suffer from medical conditions.

Non-Pharmacological Measures

The first step aims to minimize risk and ensure the safety of patients and caregivers. Aggressive behaviour not only harms caregivers, but also endangers patients by provoking aggressive responses from others. A decision on where best to care for the patient must be made, i.e., home versus hospital. Few health services have acute psychogeriatric wards equipped to care for these patients. In addition, most are cared for in medical wards where the environment is inappropriate, and staff are not adequately trained, and therefore, are unable to allocate sufficient time.

When aggressive behaviour occurs, it is important to educate caregivers, remove or alleviate triggers, maintain routines where possible, optimize medications, and treat concomitant illnesses. After any incident of aggression it is important that caregivers and health care workers discuss the episode to determine possible triggers.

Medication

Antipsychotics are often the medications of

choice for aggression. They reduce aggressive behaviour and ameliorate associated delusions and hallucinations, which are common precipitants of aggression. Empirical use of antipsychotics in the acute setting is often required. In the acute treatment phase, parenteral preparations, e.g., haloperidol 0.5-1 mg IM, may be required in combination with an oral atypical antipsychotic, e.g., risperidone 0.25 to 0.5 mg OD/BID. For subacute or chronic treatment the dose is gradually titrated to maximize symptom control with minimal side effects. Atypical antipsychotics like risperidone and olanzapine may take some time (usually weeks) to achieve full efficacy. With reduction in symptoms over time, antipsychotics may be reduced and even stopped, with caution.

Since physical aggression is strongly associated with depression[5] antidepressant medications may be used as adjuvant therapy, e.g., citalopram, sertraline, paroxetine, nefazadone or trazadone for nocturnal agitation or insomnia. It is important to recognize and treat depression as early as possible.

If, after a reasonable treatment duration, a patient does not respond satisfactorily to antipsychotics (and an antidepressant if there is a concern about depression), there are a number of ways to proceed. The next step will depend on the individual patient and the physician's preference. The range of therapeutic possibilities includes:

- Increase or decrease the dose of antipsychotic to a dose that is effective, or side effects occur.

- Try an alternative atypical antipsychotic, e.g., olanzapine, quetiapine or clozapine.
- Anti-depressants are often used as adjuvants, particularly if physical aggression is present.
- Try trazadone, if not already started, especially in patients with insomnia and nocturnal agitation.
- Add or substitute sodium valproate, commencing at a dose of 400 mg daily in divided doses and titrate slowly to response.
- Use chloral hydrate.
- Use beta-blockers.
- Use short-acting benzodiazepines.
- Try short-term estrogen or anti-androgen therapy in males. Short-term use usually avoids any significant side effects, and may be beneficial. Long-term use of estrogen may be limited by side-effects such as impotence and/or gynaecomastia in males.

The most common reason for "treatment failure" is failure to continue treatment long enough to allow for therapeutic response, because treatment may take up to 6 weeks to achieve efficacy.

Agitation[23]

Agitation includes inappropriate, non-aggressive vocal or motor activity e.g. pacing, restlessness, that frequently results from the inability of patients to express their needs and is commonly associated with confusion. There is a linear increase in agitation from dawn until dusk with an accelerated increase in the evening, referred to as **sundowning**.[6] Agitation can result from concomitant illness e.g. infection, congestive cardiac failure, inappropriate medications or dehydration. Therefore, diagnosis of "agitation secondary to dementia" should be considered as a symptom of an underlying problem. As with all dysfunctional behaviours, one must initially adopt a non-pharmacological approach to the treatment of agitation by managing the patient in a calming environment (i.e. warm temperature, reduced noise (calming music), small patient numbers if in nursing home, avoiding restraints).

Disruptive vocalizations **(calling out, screaming/crying)** occur with severe cognitive and physical impairment. Caregivers should avoid screaming or shouting back, as it only serves to reinforce this behaviour. As with an infant, crying is often a marker for a basic need such as hunger, cold, uncomfortable heat, pain, etc. Caregivers should first ensure that there is no obvious cause for distress such as pain, impaction, urinary retention, etc. Reduced auditory acuity may also promote screaming.

Once these potential causes have been ruled out and non-pharmacological measure introduced, medications such as atypical antipsychotics at low doses may be used e.g. risperidone 0.25mg BID, olanzapine 2.5mg OD or quetiapine 25mg HS. Other medications used include trazadone commencing at 25mg at night can be helpful if there is altered sleep-wake pattern. One may consider short-acting benzodiazepines (careful, they can make confusion worse). If agitation is felt to be associated with depression, commence an SSRI, e.g., sertraline 50 mg PO OD, or citalopram 10 to 20mg OD.

DYSFUNCTIONAL ACTIVITIES

Wandering

One cross-sectional study found that approximately 20% of community-dwelling people with dementia wander[20]. It is more common in men, patients with Alzheimer's disease and patients with sleep disorders . The frequency of wandering has a linear relationship with caregiver stress[19].

The factors that provoke wandering include boredom, unfamiliar surroundings, lack of exercise, anxiety and stress. Wandering becomes more dangerous to patients as functional ability declines and they become more unsteady. Nocturnal wandering and wandering in patients with reduced visual acuity also increases risk. The prevalence is reduced in more debilitated patients.

Some people wander because they are looking for something or someone; others wander for no apparent purpose. This behaviour is often repetitive if they are looking for a particular object or person. People can wander in their house, outside or in institutions. Wandering is only problematic if the person gets lost, comes to harm or disrupts others. People can wander safely in an enclosed environment if they are supervised; outdoor wandering parks in nursing homes that allow patients to wander safely can be particularly beneficial.

Nocturnal wandering is linked with sleep disorders. The risk of injury to the patient is dependent on the phase of sleep in which the wandering occurs: when it occurs during non-REM sleep, patients are more likely to injure themselves.

Wandering demonstrates the importance of maintaining a routine: a daily program of exercise for 1 to 1.5 hours will reduce the prevalence and severity of wandering in patients prone to this behaviour[21].

Newer non-benzodiazepines, for example, zolpidem, can help improve nocturnal wandering associated with insomnia and may have a normalizing effect on abnormal sleep patterns.

Sleep Disorder[7,8] (See Case 4)

Sleep disorders are common in the elderly and even more common in dementia. They may take the form of insomnia, hypersomnia or altered sleep/wake pattern. Aging reduces the overall length and depth of sleep in normal adults, by altering the production of growth hormone and melatonin, and these changes are further disrupted in dementia. In AD there is a shortening of REM sleep, multiple awakenings, and a reduction in all slow-wave sleep.

Insomnia or Altered Sleep/Wake Pattern

Insomnia may be caused by medical conditions that cause dyspnoea (especially at night), pain, anxiety, dysuria, nocturia, and even constipation. Altered sleep/wake pattern is common in dementia and is often misconstrued as insomnia because the patient is not sleeping through the night and wakes often.

Non-Pharmacological Treatment

1. Stop medications that may interfere with sleep.
2. Establish a routine. Arrange for the patient to rise, eat and retire at the same time each day. Arrange for exercise at the same time each day.
3. Avoid evening stimulation, e.g., avoid caffeine, physical activity, or watching TV late in the evening. Evening activities should be as relaxing as possible. A warm bath before bed may stimulate, rather than relax, and make matters worse.
4. Prevent daytime napping even it requires waking the patient.
5. Bright-light therapy may help.

Pharmacological Treatment

If there is associated depression, use antidepressants with mild sedative properties, e.g., paroxetine or fluvoxamine commencing at 10 mg taken in the evening.

If a sedative is required, short-term use of non-benzodiazepine hypnotics such as zopiclone 7.5 to 15.0mg qhs. The advantage of the non-benzodiazepine hypnotics is the lack of intolerance, withdrawal phenomenon or "REM rebound." These features are advantageous if long-term use of these medications is required. If one uses traditional benzodiazepines, they should be short-acting, for example, lorazepam 0.5 to 1.0 mg at night and used for a short duration.

Chloral hydrate has been widely used in the treatment of insomnia in the elderly. The main concern is overdose and cross-tolerance with alcohol. It is given as 0.5 to 1.0 grams and has a rapid onset of action. Trazodone (a tetracyclic antidepressant) is a very useful sedative that may also reduce some DBDs such as agitation and aggression. A strategy that is sometimes adopted is to alternate sedatives every five days or so to avoid tolerance and dependency. It also provides information on which medication worked best. It is essential that caregivers get sleep because if they continue to lose sleep, they will burn out.

Apathy[9,10]

Closely linked with depression but nonetheless a distinct neuropsychiatric entity, apathy occurs in about one fifth of demented patients. It occurs more frequently in patients with frontal lobe dementia or frontal lobe-related cognitive deficits in AD. Apathy is more closely related to lower cognitive function than depression. Loss of interest in activities may result from loss of ability to participate in those activities, as happens in retirement from work without other interests to take up free time.

Distinguishing between apathy as a consequence of dementia, and depression, is a difficult diagnostic challenge. Investigations such as single positron emission computerized tomography (SPECT) (abnormal in frontotemporal dementia), MRI and/or EEG (abnormal in dementia, normal in depression) can help to resolve this clinical dilemma.

Apathy with dementia is a difficult symptom to treat. Management involves removing potential causes, then treating with antidepressants and cholinergic drugs. The first step is to remove drugs, if possible, that may cause apathy, e.g., sedatives, anxiolytics or many cardiac drugs (B-blockers, amiodarone, digoxin etc.), and rule out other causes such as hypothyroidism or Parkinson's disease. Attempts should be made to socially stimulate apathetic patients by getting them involved in activities that previously interested them.

Antidepressants such as desipramine, nortryptiline, venlafaxine, sertraline or low dose fluoxetine (5 to 10 mg) are the most widely used medications for apathy. When apathy occurs in the setting of depression and does not respond to drugs, ECT may be considered. Apathy associated with dementia (not associated with a major depressive disorder) may not respond to antidepressants. In these patients cholinesterase inhibitors may have a beneficial effect[21]. Methylphenidate 2.5 mg or tea may be also tried.

Eating Disorders[11,13,14]

Anorexia

A common problem in AD, anorexia causes concern because it is often associated with weight loss. Forgetting to eat is a major problem among demented people. Although, strictly speaking, not a DBD, anorexia leads to malnutrition and has a negative impact on general health. It occurs most commonly in demented people who live alone without daily supervision. Malnutrition can aggravate DBD and is preventable in most cases.

Many speculative theories have been proposed to account for anorexia and weight loss, including atrophy of the medial temporal cortex. Interventions that educate caregivers in nutritional requirements, and approaches to encourage eating and improve social supports (such as Meals on Wheels) are helpful. Increased caregiver burden increases the risk of inadequate nutrition. Weight loss secondary to AD is a diagnosis of exclusion as there is a high prevalence of other causes of weight loss in this age group. The extent to which clinicians should seek other causes depends on each individual's circumstances.

Pharmacological approaches include treating medical causes of anorexia. Dronabinol has been studied in a small number of patients with AD and is beneficial in the treatment of anorexia and other dysfunctional behaviours. There is insufficient evidence at present to recommend it for routine use.[12] Anorexia can also be a vegetative sign of depression, either with or without dementia.

Hyperphagia

In dementia, hyperphagia occurs in approximately 23% of patients, usually in the moderate stages of the disease[11]. The most florid examples of hyperphagia are seen in frontotemporal dementia, often with a hyperoral element where patients repeatedly put non-edible objects in their mouths. This condition often alternates with periods of anorexia. Hyperphagia does not always mean that these patients have adequate nutritional intake. Some patients may have excessive caloric intake, resulting in weight gain which may compromise mobility and dependency.

Simple measures such as giving frequent small healthy snacks instead of large meals may be effective.

Hoarding

About 25% of demented patients hoard[22] . It is not always clear why they do this, but it may be a feature of an underlying obsessive trait or a feature of paranoia. There is no specific treatment so a simple initial measure is to determine if there is a particular reason why the patient is hoarding. Some patients hide money or belongings because they are unfamiliar with their surroundings, and reassurance may be all that is required. SSRIs like paroxetine may be effective.

Depending on the clinical circumstances (i.e., how much of a problem hoarding represents and whether it is a consequence of paranoid delusions) a low dose of an antipsychotic may be considered.

DYSFUNCTIONAL PERCEPTIONS

Hallucinations[15,16,17]

Hallucinations occur in 12 to 53% of patients with AD.[15] "True" hallucinations need to be distinguished from sensory misperceptions that result from patients' reduced ability to interpret their surroundings: for example, when a patient looks in the mirror and sees a stranger looking back, or fails to recognize a family member or friend. Reduced auditory acuity also makes sensory interpretation more difficult.

Visual hallucinations are strongly associated with disorders of the visual system, older age and female sex (in patients with AD). They are the most common type of hallucination and occur in all forms of dementia, but more commonly in Lewy body dementia, where 48% of patients experience them. They may also be provoked by dopaminergic and anticholinergic medications.

In Lewy body dementia, the hallucinations do not always distress the patient and are sometimes accepted as being normal and non-intrusive. An example of this is a gentleman who saw performing circus animals in his living room and considered them entertaining. However, it was distressing to the caregiver, especially when visitors called.

Hallucinations need to be problematic to warrant treatment. In some patients, treatment may be neither necessary nor appropriate, given the sensitivity of patients with Lewy body dementia to antipsychotics.

In cases where treatment is required, we would recommend risperidone 0.25 mg hs increasing very slowly (every week or so) to a maximum of 2 mg/day, with utmost caution. In patients with Lewy body dementia and Parkinson's disease quetiapine is most commonly used, starting at 12.5-25mg at night increasing slowly up to about 100mg/day. In Lewy body dementia we would recommend anticholinesterases as first-line therapy for the treatment of hallucinations.

Drugs that can cause Hallucinations/Delusions

• Prednisone
• Anticholinergic
• Serontonergic antidepressants
• Dopaminergics
• NSAIDs

Delusions[15,16,17]

Between 10 and 73% of patients with AD have delusions at some time in the course of their disease[17]. Delusions occur in all forms of dementia but are more common in Lewy body dementia and Parkinson's disease. It is our experience that they are also more common in Alzheimer's disease than Vascular Dementia.

Paranoid delusions are the most common. Paranoid delusions place caregivers at risk when patients believe that the caregiver is unfaithful, plotting against them or fail to recognize them and believe them to be strangers.

Delusions themselves never require treatment. They are only treated if they cause distress to patients or caregivers, or put either at risk. If delusions distress either patients (e.g., thinks she has cancer and is going to die) or caregivers (e.g., thinks mother is still alive and keeps wanting to visit her), or precipitate behaviour that puts either at risk (e.g., thinks wife is having affair with postman and is threatening to kill both), start risperidone 0.25 to 0.5 mg HS. Risperidone may be increased every 5 days or so in 0.25 to 0.5 mg increments until delusions resolve. SSRI antidepressants can be used if the delusions are suspected to be related to depression (for example, the patient may believe that he or she has cancer, or that all his or her money is gone). Anticholinesterases may also reduce delusions in Lewy body dementia and AD, and should be used.

It is also important to assess for suicidal ideation in delusional patients.

CLINICAL GEMS

- Behaviour needs to be dysfunctional before it requires treatment.
- Therapy usually takes days and often weeks to exert a clinical effect—avoid increasing doses in a short period of time in an effort to achieve a "quick fix".
- DBD is usually not cured, but rather improved, and this should be reflected in the clinical goals.
- Start low and go slow. Rule of thumb—commence medications in the elderly at half the recommended starting dose for younger adults.

Chapter 9

CASE EXAMPLES

CASE 1: "I WANT TO GO HOME!"

Miss R., a 79-year-old woman, was diagnosed with Alzheimer's disease (AD) 18 months ago when she presented with short-term memory loss, and was making mistakes in her finances, e.g., wrong names and amounts on cheques (which was very unusual for her). Neighbours and friends had commented with some surprise on her recent loss of personal hygiene because she had always been fastidiously clean and tidy person.

Miss R. had lived on her own for over 50 years and was well known because she owned and managed a successful interior decorating company. Although likeable, she was independent, headstrong and at times, difficult. Throughout her life she had remained active, taking regular walks each evening and had a keen interest in gardening.

Six months ago, Miss R. moved to a retirement home, where she appeared to settle in well and took walks regularly in the evening. One month ago she developed a urinary tract infection and became more confused at this time. After this, she began wandering. She frequently went missing and was usually found roaming about the streets, apparently lost. When asked where she was going, she would reply, "I'm going home, I need to get there," and often became argumentative and agitated but never aggressive when people tried to redirect her. Recently the wandering had become more problematic because she had gone out at night.

Her family physician prescribed haloperidol 0.5 mg at night. Her wandering didn't stop but she did become more unsteady and on one occasion was found at the end of the garden, lying on the ground.

On assessment, her Standardized Mini Mental State Examination (SMMSE) was 20/30.

Causative Theory

This case demonstrates the interplay between different causative theories. Miss R. has had a change in her environment, with which she initially coped well. However, as her capacity to cope with stressful situations became more impaired (e.g., by the change in routine and co-morbid urinary tract infection) her coping mechanisms were overwhelmed. The urge to go walking, a routine for many years, was not rationalized appropriately, resulting in poor judgment, so she went for walks at night. Because of impaired short-term recall, Miss R. suddenly found herself lost and was unsure where she was going. She presumed that she was going home and when approached by people she did not recognize, she was frightened and agitated. Having been formerly independent and head-strong, she insisted that she was fully aware of what she was doing and where she was going.

ABCDE CHECKLIST
(Clinical Tool 1, Chapter 5)

ADL Activities of Daily Living	Miss R. is dependent in instrumental ADL (IADL) e.g. finances, driving, shopping and requires minimal assistance with washing, grooming and toileting. She dresses and feeds independently.
Behaviour	Activity: she has been wandering lately at night and she has a disrupted sleep-wake pattern. Response: she became agitated when questioned about her behaviour and when people tried to redirect her. No aggressive behaviour.
Cognition	SMMSE score is 20/30. Short-term memory loss with disorientation to time and place.
Depression	No evidence of changes in vegetative signs (except for sleep) or mood.
Effects on Caregiver	The staff members in the retirement home are concerned for Miss R.'s safety.

Five-step Approach to DBD
(Clinical Tool 4, Chapter 5)

DESCRIBE THE BEHAVIOUR What the person does exactly? How often? How long does it last? Who is it problem for?	She wanders about the home and grounds every evening. She may wander for 1 hour or more providing she doesn't get lost. It is of concern to the nursing staff and it is putting the patient at considerable risk.
DESCRIBE TRIGGERS AND CONSEQUENCES	Change of environment Urinary tract infection An alteration in her routine with increased risk of falling and injury
DEVELOP REALISTIC GOALS	Ensure safety Restore and maintain routine Wandering will not stop but it can be supervised with appropriate timing Stop antipsychotic
DEVELOP A CAREPLAN	Arrange regular supervised walks Increase activities e.g., gardening Wandering Patient Registry
EVALUATE TREATMENT	Review in outpatients in 1 month or sooner if there is any deterioration Re-assess ABCDE of dementia Review medications

Goals of Treatment

Inappropriate Goals

It is inappropriate to believe that Miss R.'s behaviour can be treated with medications alone. The introduction of antipsychotics has already put this woman at increased risk. Barriers in the form of medications or physical retraints will only result in harm to the patient with loss of dignity, freedom, function and autonomy. This approach to treatment, i.e., increasing antipsychotics and other forms of restraints, will stop the wandering behaviour but the costs of increased sedation and impaired mobility are too high a price to pay for her.

Realistic Goals

1. Ensure safety. Stop antipsychotics, which are making her unsteady and not improving the behaviour.

2. Understand what is causing the behaviour. The behaviour is a dysfunctional routine and can only be effectively treated if attempts are made to restore a normal/functional routine. We advised daily walks for 40 minutes to 1 hour.

3. Miss R.'s ability to learn new routines and adapt to changes in her environment has

become increasingly impaired and it will take time for her to re-adjust to proposed changes.

4. Maintain personal liberties, e.g., allow her to choose clothes, food, regular walks. She has been a fiercely independent woman through- out her life and every effort should be made to maintain this independence without putting her at risk.

5. It is unlikely that this behaviour will fully resolve. In this case Miss R. will most likely continue to occasionally wander the corridors but can do so safely if supervised.

Care Plan

Take Miss R. for a supervised walk every day with family, friend, volunteer or staff member. En- sure that the same route is followed every day. If she does wander, it is likely that she will take this path and find it easier to return home—she will also be easier to find because if she does wander she will most likely use this familiar route out of habit. We also sub- mitted her name and photograph to the Wandering Patients Registry at the local Alzheimer's Society.

CASE 2: A Circus in the Living Room

Mr Y. is a 72-year-old gentleman with a two-year history of progressive memory loss. His wife feels that the memory loss is more obvious some days than others. She has also noticed that he has "slowed down" in the past year and appears unsteady on his feet. He has had no falls, yet.

Recently, he had visual hallucinations where he saw people in the house but his wife did not see anybody. At times he found this distressing. In the last 2 months, he has been seeing small animals in the house and believes that they are playing but they do not talk to him. He does not appear to be distressed by them but his wife has some concern because he points them out to visitors, who find it unsettling.

ABCDE CHECKLIST
(Clinical Tool 1, Chapter 5)

ADL Activities of Daily Living	Mr Y. is independent in basic ADL and is dependent for IADL. He has not looked after the couple's finances or driven in 18 months. There is some concern because of his unsteady gait and risk of falls.
Behaviour	<u>Perceptions:</u> Visual hallucinations are not distressing to the patient. He had delusions previously but they have since resolved.
Cognition	SMMSE score is 24/30.
Depression	No evidence of vegetative signs or mood disturbance.
Effects on Caregiver	The caregiver is concerned by this behaviour although it does not affect the patient.

Five-step Approach to DBD
(Clinical Tool 4, Chapter 5)

DESCRIBE THE BEHAVIOUR What the person does exactly? How often? How long does it last? Who is it a problem for?	Visual hallucinations Two to three time in the past 2 months 20 minutes to 1 hour Caregiver
DESCRIBE TRIGGERS AND CONSEQUENCES	No obvious triggers Distress to caregiver
DEVELOP REALISTIC GOALS	Cessation or improvement in frequency of visual hallucinations
DEVELOP A CAREPLAN	Educate and reassure caregiver Commence anticholinesterase
EVALUATE TREATMENT	Reviewed in outpatients after 3 months - improvement in symptoms

Clinical Impression

On examination, Mr Y. had bradykinesia, loss of normal arm swing, facial masking and increased tone bilaterally. He was noted to have a significant drop in his systolic blood pressure upon standing (160/80 mmHg lying; 110/60 mmHg standing). This man was diagnosed as probable Lewy body dementia.

Care Plan

Mr and Mrs Y. were informed of the likely diagnosis of probable Lewy body dementia. They were reassured that the visual hallucinations are a well-recognized feature of Lewy body dementia and that it may respond to anticholinesterases, a new treatment for dementia. The goals of treatment were discussed. The couple were informed that it may take weeks for symptoms to improve.

Mr Y. was started on donepezil or rivastigmine. Upon review after 6 weeks, the frequency and duration of his hallucinations had improved. He was tolerating the new medication well. The dose was increased and fludrocortisone 0.1 mg OD was commenced to treat his postural hypotension. Other potential approaches to the treatment of postural hypotension are the following: midodrine, phenylephrine, clonidine or dihydroergotamine, which vasoconstrict vessels; prostaglandin-synthase inhibitors that prevent vasodilation, like indomethacin and fluoribiprofen; and the dopamine receptor-blocker metoclopropamide plus domperidone and/or propranolol. A beta-2 adrenoreceptor blocker that prevents vasodilation may also be used.

CASE 3: THE STRANGER IN THE MIRROR

Mr Jones, a 68-year old, was diagnosed with dementia four years ago. He has other medical problems. He relies on his wife to help him with most aspects of basic ADL care, i.e., needs supervision bathing and dressing, and has occasional episodes of urinary incontinence. His wife says that he cannot recognize himself in the mirror and often stands in front of the mirror in the bathroom for 20 minutes talking to his own image. At times he becomes annoyed because the person in the mirror will not answer him. He also talks to his reflection in the oven door. She is able to cope with this behaviour at home but she is concerned when he talks to his reflection in shop windows and car doors. When this happens she is unable to stop his "conversations." She is unable to leave him alone in the house and feels trapped because she can't go out alone anymore.

ABCDE CHECKLIST
(Clinical Tool 1, Chapter 5)

ADL Activities of Daily Living	Mr Jones is only able to feed himself. He needs supervision or assistance with all other ADLs. Mrs Jones would benefit from a community nurse and a health care aid to help with ADL care, e.g., showering and dressing.
Behaviour	The DBD has been identified. Mrs Jones has suggested some strategies to deal with the problem herself. An anti-cholinesterase may be tried
Cognition	His SMMSE score is 15/30.
Depression	Mr Jones cannot complete the GDS (Geriatric Depression Scale) but there is no evidence that he is depressed.
Effects on Caregiver	Mrs Jones completes the Zarit burden scale and this shows considerable stress.

Five-step Approach to DBD
(Clinical Tool 4, Chapter 5)

DESCRIBE THE BEHAVIOUR What the person does exactly? How often? How long does it last? Who is it problem for?	He interprets his image in the mirror as being a stranger It occurs every day It is a problem for both patient and caregiver
DESCRIBE TRIGGERS AND CONSEQUENCES	All reflective objects distress to the patient
DEVELOP REALISTIC GOALS	Avoid triggers Educate and reassure caregiver Refer to Alzheimer's society for education and support
DEVELOP A CAREPLAN	Remove or cover all reflective objects in the house Patient to attend day-care centre Anti-cholinesterase
EVALUATE TREATMENT	Review in Outpatients in 1 month Assess ABCDE of dementia Review medications

Care Plan

- Mrs. Jones will either remove or cover all reflective objects in the house.
- She will ask her daughter or a home care worker to come and stay with Mr. Jones when she needs to go out shopping.
- The health care team will organize a community nurse and/or health care aid to come to assist Mr. Jones with ADL care, e.g., showering and dressing.
- Respite will be organized to give Mrs. Jones a break from the stress of caring for her husband.
- The team provides Mrs. Jones with a full explanation about the DBD and reassures her that it will probably resolve over time.
- Mr. Jones will attend a day-care centre one day a week to give his wife a break.
- Try a cholinesterase inhibitor.
- Mrs. Jones will contact the Alzheimer's Society to learn more about the disease, get educational resourses and/or join a support group.

CASE 4: UP AT NIGHT

Mr H. is a 72-year-old man who was initially assessed at clinic 6 months ago when he was diagnosed as probable AD. He also has type 2 diabetes mellitus that is well controlled with oral antiglycemics.

Caregiver Interview

His wife, his only caregiver, states: "He's not sleeping, doctor. He's up all night walking around the house, rummaging in the kitchen. I'm exhausted. I've had no sleep for the last week because he keeps waking me up!"

When did this start?

"It began about 2 months ago when he started waking up in the middle of the night coughing and spluttering. At first he stayed awake for about an hour before he settled back to sleep. He used to be really confused when it happened and he never remembered it afterwards, but I guess he was very tired. I rang our family physician and he gave me a prescription for a sleeping tablet that only made things worse."

In what way?

"The sleeping pill made him more confused during the night and it took him longer to settle. He was very sleepy in the morning and started to sleep to lunchtime, which suited me fine because it gave me a chance to do the housework. Normally, his friends called and took him out for lunch and I had used that time to get the housework done. But they stopped taking him because he started falling asleep during lunch."

So what happened then?

"When things didn't improve after the week I brought him back to the doctor. He examined him and told me that he had fluid on the chest and started him on a fluid tablet and another pill called Ramipril. His breathing improved but he is still not getting any sleep at night."

How much sleep does he get during the day?

"About 3 hours in the morning and maybe 60 to 90 minutes in the afternoon. At night he sleeps for 3 hours and wakes at 3a.m."

Does he get agitated?

"No, but I find that I am getting more cross with him because I am not getting any sleep at all now."

Key Points

1. If the trigger to this problem had been recognized in time it may not have escalated into such a difficult situation.

2. The original complaint was that the patient wasn't sleeping, but in fact the patient was getting an adequate amount of sleep each day. The sleep routine at night had been disrupted by daytime napping. This routine was accepted at first by the spouse because it afforded her time to do her housework. The patient has day/night reversal. His sleep routine has changed and he is still sleeping about 6 to 7 hours per day.

3. This case illustrates the importance of maintaining a routine. The cessation of going to lunch with his friends has had an impact on his night-time waking.

ABCDE CHECKLIST
(Clinical Tool 1, Chapter 5)

ADL Activities of Daily Living	Independent ADL, dependent for IADL.
Behaviour	<u>Activity</u> Up at night, sleeping during the day, day/night reversal.
Cognition	SMMSE score is 21/30.
Depression	No depression or vegetative signs other than sleep disturbance.
Effects on Caregiver	Caregiver exhausted from sleep deprivation.

Five-step Approach to DBD
(Clinical Tool 4, Chapter 5)

DESCRIBE THE BEHAVIOUR What the person does exactly? How often? How long does it last? Who is it problem for?	Wandering at night, insomnia; daytime somnolence Every night Three to four hours Patient and caregiver
DESCRIBE TRIGGERS AND CONSEQUENCES	Cardiac failure with PND (paroxysmal nocturnal dyspnoea) Insomnia for patient and caregiver Substantial increase in caregiver burden - "I get angry much easier", "I'm exhausted."
DEVELOP REALISTIC GOALS	Treat cardiac failure Restore regular sleeping pattern Improve aid services to caregiver Alzheimer's Society
DEVELOP A CAREPLAN	Up during the day with day-care centre and activities with regular exercise Sedation at night for 10 days to help restore wake/sleep pattern
EVALUATE TREATMENT	Review in outpatients clinic in 1 month

Care Plan

Environment

Avoid daytime sleeping, including "catnaps." Encourage his friends to take Mr H. to lunch again each day. Include morning or afternoon walks, gently at first in view of the cardiac failure. Other simple measures include avoiding caffeine, especially in the evening, and taking meals at regular times. Make the caregiver aware that these simple measures, although often difficult in the short-term, will work eventually. Increasing help in the home, even for a short while, will help to avoid/reduce caregiver burnout. Consider day-care centre.

Medical

Appropriate treatment of his cardiac failure with attention to timing of medications, e.g., diuretics taken in the morning and nitrates at night is key. If required, use sedatives like zopiclone, trazodone or chloral hydrate in the short term to re-establish sleeping at night. Medications that are most commonly used for nocturnal sedation particularly benzodiazepines may also contribute to nocturnal confusion and increase the risk of falling. If the patient is sleeping during the day then this can allow the caregiver a break, but escalation of the insomnia at night leads to caregiver burnout, early institutionalization and/or hospital admission.

CASE 5: THE IMAGINARY LOVER

Mr Simpson is 75 years old and has had two minor strokes in recent years. He has a history of high blood pressure, prostate cancer, diabetes and peripheral vascular disease. He complains of burning in his feet, which is worse at night and keeps him awake. After the first stroke he has had difficulty walking and since the second stroke 2 years ago, his wife has noticed progressive memory loss.

At his first memory assessment 12 months ago, he scored 18/30 on the SMMSE. His brain scan showed two small strokes deep in the brain. He failed a driving assessment last year and blamed his wife for this.

In the last 3 months his behaviour has changed. He gets angry with his wife, accuses her of having affairs and scheming against him. He shouts at her and lately has been waving his fist and threatening her.

Now his wife is scared and says she can't cope much longer because:
- He is very prone to temper outbursts
- He frequently raises his fist to her in a threatening way, but has never hit her
- He follows her around the house
- He accuses her of having a boyfriend and lying to him
- Sometimes at night he tells her she had better leave the house, or he will kill her

- Last night he went to bed with a two-foot long metal pipe.

ABCDE CHECKLIST
(Clinical Tool 1, Chapter 5)

ADL Activities of Daily Living	Mr S. is no longer able to drive, manage finances or help with shopping. He needs assistance with dressing, grooming and bathing. He walks with a cane.
Behaviour	Mr S. has three identifiable dysfunctional behaviours : • <u>Dysfunctional response</u> — aggression and agitation (shouts and waves his fists at his wife) • <u>Dysfunctional perceptions</u>—delusion of infidelity. • <u>Dysfunctional routine</u>—up at night. • Mrs S. completes the Dysfunctional Behaviour in Dementia Rating Instrument (DBDRI, see Chapter 5) to quantify the problems and their effect on her.

Cognition	Mr S. scores 13/30 on the SMMSE. This shows further deterioration in the previous 12 months.
Depression	There is no evidence of significant mood disorder. Mr S scores 3/15 on the depression scale, which is not suggestive of depression. Note, however, that as cognitive function deteriorates, the depression scores become less reliable and valid.
Effects on Caregiver	Mrs S. completes the Zarit burden scale, which shows considerable burden. She does not know how to cope with these episodes and is afraid that her husband will harm her when she is asleep. She scores 16/30 on the Geriatric Depression scale. Her case is discussed with he family physician and she is commenced on Citalopram 20mg OD.

Five-step Approach to DBD
(Clinical Tool 4, Chapter 5)

DESCRIBE THE BEHAVIOUR What the person does exactly? How often? How long does it last? Who is it problem for?	Accuses wife of infidelity Follows her everywhere Temper outbursts waving fists in air up at night for three to four hours Patient and caregiver
DESCRIBE TRIGGERS AND CONSEQUENCES	He sees me talking to the grocer Behaviour reinforced by wife arguing back Mrs. S. has become angry, frustrated and frightened and depressed
DEVELOP REALISTIC GOALS	Treat paranoid ideation Control pain in feet Ensure safety of caregiver and patient
DEVELOP A CAREPLAN	Modify environment Remove weapons Educate Mrs. S. Alzheimer's society Commence risperidone 0.5mg HS or olanzapine 2.5mg HS Commence analgesics Commence donepezil 5mg OD or rivastigmine 1.5mg BID
EVALUATE TREATMENT	Reviewed in outpatients weekly

Care Plan

The wife is clearly at risk and this problem needs immediate attention. The management plan is put in place by the health care team based on the information obtained from the assessment.

Current Medications

Lorazepam 1 mg TID prn

> For anxiety/agitation

Metformin 250 mg three times a day

> For diabetes

Glyburide 10 mg daily

> For diabetes

Digoxin 125 μg daily

> For heart rhythm

Aspirin 325 mg daily

> To prevent stroke

Diclofenac 50 mg three times daily

> For foot pain

Atenolol 25 mg daily

> For blood pressure

Management setting

The decision to manage this case at home or in hospital will depend on the degree of risk to the patient and caregiver if we keep him in the home. Mrs S. says that she wants to keep her husband at home as long as possible and is prepared to try any new medications and suggestions to manage the aggression. She has also agreed to take an anti-depressant prescribed by her family physician.

Non-Pharmacological Management

1. Maintain calm environment using well-lit room with soothing music. Avoid conversation that may promote agitation, e.g., driving privileges. Avoid arguments when he starts talking about driving again by changing the subject or distracting him. Take the car out of the driveway so that he is not constantly reminded of it. Use calming words and touch to respond to his emotions rather than logic or explanations.

2. Maintain Routine. This may prove difficult as caregivers often try to avoid public places and contact with other people because of fear or embarrassment. Daily walks or day-care centre may relieve the stress on Mrs. S. will get community nursing, family and homemakers to come in to help her, especially in the short term.

3. Mrs. S to contact the Alzheimer's society for education and support.

Pharmacological Treatment

1. Start risperidone 0.5 mg at night, 0.25 mg BID or olanzapine 2.5mg hs. Risperidone is used for delusions and aggression. The dose of risperidone will need to be reviewed at least weekly to bring the problem under immediate control.

2. Start donepezil 5 mg, rivastigmine 1.5 mg BID or galantamine 4mg BID. This may help memory and behaviour. The main side effects are nausea, vomiting and/or diarrhea. The dose should be increased in 4 weeks if the drug is tolerated.

3. Check digoxin level and reduce digoxin dose to 62.5 μg. Digoxin can cause confusion because it has some anticholinergic effects. The lower dose is probably sufficient for the cardiac problem. Get a community nurse to monitor heart rate because the donepezil and digoxin may exacerbate his bradycardia.

4. Start trazodone 25 to 50 mg or Zopiclone 7.5 to 15mg at night for sleep. Features of depression should be actively sought.

5. Start Mrs. S on an anti-depressant.

Additional Considerations

1. If there is a clinical suspicion of depression, commence an antidepressant, e.g., paroxetine 20 mg PO qhs. Paroxetine is chosen because it is sedating and although it has some anticholinergic effects, it will also treat anxiety. Another choice here might be sertraline 50 mg OD or citalopram 10 mg OD or nefazadone 50 mg BID.

2. Pain is a trigger of dysfunctional behaviour and it needs to be controlled. This will also promote a good night's sleep. The foot pain is most likely from diabetic neuropathy. We recommend appropriate foot care and gabapentin orally for neuropathic pain if simple analgesics are ineffective. Gabapentin is not given on this visit because we are starting risperidone, donepezil and possibly trazodone now. At the next visit, we may try gabapentin if these measures and/or simple analgesics are ineffective.

3. Contact community nursing and consider community psychiatric services for follow-up in the community.

4. Review all other medications.

5. Review the situation by phone daily for 1 week.

6. Review in clinic in 1 week.

7. Arrange for attendance at a day-care centre for activities when behaviour is under control.

8. Arrange respite for Mr S. in a dementia facility as soon as possible to give Mrs S. a break.

AUTHORS

1. **Martin O'Donnell** MB, MRCP(I), a fellow in Geriatric medicine at the Geriatric Research Group and Memory Clinic, McMaster University, Ontario, Canada. Qualified from University College Cork, Ireland in 1994. He had worked in clinical geriatric medicine for three years prior to joining the Geriatric Research Group in Jan 2000. Working alongside Dr. D.W. Molloy, he has developed a research interest in the behavioural and psychological symptoms of dementia.

2. **D. William Molloy**, MB, MRCP(I), FRCP(C) is a Geriatrician who specializes in treating patients with dementia, particularly Alzheimer's disease. He has worked with the elderly and their families for more than twenty years. He has gained extensive practical and theoretical experience in this field. Dr. Molloy is Director of the Geriatric Research Group and Memory Clinic at the Hamilton Health Sciences Corporation, Henderson Division. He is a Professor of Medicine, McMaster University, Hamilton. Dr. Molloy is the author of *Let Me Decide*, *Set Me Free*, *Vital Choices*, *What Are We Going to do Now?*, *The Fine Detail*, *Alzheimer's disease*, (co-written with Dr. Paul Caldwell), *How do You Say?*,*The SMMSE User's Guide*, *Thirteen Months of Sunshine*, *Let Me Pass Gently and Capacity to Decide*.

3. **Kiran Rabheru** MD BSc FRCPC, a geriatric psychiatrist, originally moved from Tanzania (East Africa) to Ottawa, Ontario, where he graduated from high school in 1972. At the University of Western Ontario (UWO), in London, Ontario, he completed an Honours BSc. in Microbiology & Immunology (1976) and an MD (1980) followed by a rotating internship. After five years of general practice, he returned to UWO and completed his residency in Psychiatry in 1990. He has obtained his FRCP in Canada, board certification in Psychiatry and in Geriatric Psychiatry in the USA. Although his main area of interest since 1990 has been Geriatric Psychiatry, he maintains a keen interest in primary care and is a Certificant of the College of Family Medicine of Canada.

Currently, he is medical co-leader of the Geriatric Psychiatry Program at London/ St. Thomas Psychiatric Hospital and Associate Professor (part-time) at UWO, Department of Psychiatry. He spends much of his time caring for the elderly who suffer from dementia, mood and psychotic disorders.

REFERENCES

CHAPTER 1

1. Canadian Study of Health and Aging Working Group. Canadian study of health and aging: study methods and prevalence of dementia. Canadian Medical Association Journal 1994;150:899-913.

2. Small G, Rabins P, Barry P, Buckholtz N, DeKosky S, Ferris S et al. Daignosis and treatment of Alzheimer's disease and related disorders. Consensus statement of the American Association for Geriatric Psychiatry, the Alzheimer's Association, and the American Geriatric Society. JAMA 1997 Oct 22-29:278(16):1363-71

3. Clyburn LD, Stones MJ, Hadjistavropoulos T, Tuokko H. Predicting caregiver burden and depression in Alzheimer's disease. J Gerontol B Psychol Sci Soc Sci 2000;55:S2-13.

4. Bedard M, Molloy DW, Pedlar D, Lever JA, Stones MJ. 1997 IPA/Bayer Research Awards in Psychogeriatrics. Associations between dysfunctional behaviours, gender, and burden in spousal caregivers of cognitively impaired older adults. Int Psychogeriatr 1997 Sep;9(3):277-90

5. Balestreri L, Grossberg A, Grossberg GT. Behavioural and psychological symptoms of dementia as a risk factor for nursing home placement. International Psychogeriatrics 2000;12[Suppl. 1]:59-62.

6. Schulz R, Beach SR. Caregiving as a risk factor for mortality: the caregiver health effects study. JAMA 1999 Dec15; 282(23):2215-9

Other Reading

O'Connor DW. Epidemiology of behavioral and psychological symptoms of dementia Internatonal psychogeriatrics 2000;12[Suppl. 1]: 41-45.

Burns A. Behavioral and psychological symptoms of dementia and caregiver burden International Psychogeriatrics 2000;12[Suppl. 1]:347-350.

CHAPTER 3

1. Clyburn LD, Stones MJ, Hadjistavropoulos T, Tuokko H. Predicting caregiver burden and depression in Alzheimer's disease. J Gerontol B Psychol Sci Soc Sci 2000;55:S2-13.

2. Bedard M, Molloy DW, Pedlar D, Lever JA, Stones MJ. 1997 IPA/Bayer Research Awards in Psychogeriatrics. Associations between dysfunctional behaviours, gender, and burden in spousal caregivers of cognitively impaired older adults. Int Psychogeriatr 1997 Sep;9(3):277-90

3. Cohen-Mansfield J, Billig N. Agitated behaviours in the elderly I. A conceptual review. Journal of the American Geriatrics Society 1986;34:711-721.

4. O'Donnell BF, Drachman DA, Barnes HJ, Petreson KE, Swearer JM, Lew RA. Incontinence and troublesome behaviours predict institutionalisation in dementia. J Geriatr Psychiatry Neurol 1992 Jan-Mar; 5(1):45-52

5. Meins W. Impact of personality on behavioral and psychological symptoms of dementia. International Psychogeriatrics 2000;12[Suppl.1]:107-109.

6. Swearer JM, Hoople NE, Kane KJ, Drachmann DA. Predicting abberant behavior in Alzheimer's disease. Neuropsychiatry, Neuropsychology and Behavioral Neurology 1996;9:163-170.

7. Forstl H. Neuropathology of behavioral and psychological symptoms of dementia. International Psychogeriatrics 2000;12[Suppl.1]:77-81.

8. Mega MS, Lee L, Dinov ID, Mishkin F, Toga AW, Cummings JL. Cerebral correlates of psychotic symptoms in Alzheimer's disease. J Neurol Neursurg Psychiatry 200 Aug;69(2):167-71

9. Kirby M, Lawlor BA. Biologic markers and neurochemical correlates of agitation and psychosis in dementia. J Geriatr Psychiatry Neurol 1995 Oct;8 Suppl 1:S2-7.

10. Tariot PN. Treatment of agitation in dementia. J Clin Psychiatry 1999;60 [suppl8]:11-20.

Other Reading

Dyck G. Management of Geriatric Behavior Problems. Psychiatr Clin North Am 1997;20:165-180.

Eriksson S. Impact of the environment on behavioral and psychological symptoms of dementia. International Psychogeriatrics 2000;12[Suppl. 1]:89-91.

Jost BC, Grossberg GT. The evolution of psychiatric symptoms in Alzheimer's disease: A natural history study. Journal of the American Geriatric Society 1996 Sep;44(9):1078-81

Swearer JM, Drachman DA, O'Donnell BF, Mitchel AL. Troublesome and destructive behaviours in dementia. Journal of the American Geriatrics Society 1988;36:784-790.

Cohen-Mansfield J, Marx M, Rosenthal A. A description of agitation in a nursing home. Journal of Gerontology 1989;44:M77-M84.

Deutsch L, Rovner B. Agitation and other noncognitive abnormalities in Alzheimer's disease. The Psychiatric Clinics of North America 1991;14:341-351.

Reisberg B, Borenstein J, Salob S, et al. Behavioural symptoms in Alzheimer's disease: Phenomenology and treatment. Journal of Clinical Psychiatry 1987;5:9-15.

Cohen-Mansfield J, Billig N. Agitated behaviors in the elderly II. Preliminary results in the cognitively deteriorated. Journal of the American Geriatrics Society 1986;34:722-727.

CHAPTER 4

1. Kaye JA Diagnostic challenges in dementia. Neurology 1998 Jul;51[Suppl 1]; discussion S65-7.

2. Diagnosis and treatment of alzheimer's disease and related disorders: Consensus statement of the American Association for Geriatric Psychiatry, the Alzheimer's Association, and the American Geriatrics Society. JAMA 1997;278:1363-1371.

3. Vascular Dementia Supplement Review Alzheimer's disease and associated disorders. 1999;13[Suppl. 3]:.

4. McKeith IG, Galasko D, Kosaka K, Perry EK, Dickson DW. Consensus guidelines for the clinical and pathologic diagnosis of dementia with Lewy bodies (DLB): Report of the consortium on DLB international workshop. Neurology 1998;47:1113-1124.

5. Aarsland D, Larsen JP, Lim NG, Janvin C, Karlsen K, Tandberg E, Cummings JL Range of neuropsychiatric disturbances in patients with Parkinson's disease. J Neurol Neurosurg Psychiatry 1999 Oct;67(4):492-6

6. Mendez MF, Perryman KM, Miller BL, Cummings JL. Behavioral differences between frontotemporal dementia and Alzheimer's disease: a comparison on the BEHAVE-AD rating scale. Int Psychogeriatr 1998 Jun;10(2):155-62

7. Devanand DP, Sano M, Tang MX, Taylor S, Gurland BJ et al. Depressed mood and the incidence of Alzheimer's disease in the elderly living in the community. Archives of General Psychiatry 1996;53:175-182.

8. Allen H, Jolley D, Comish J, Burns A. Depression in dementia: a study of mood in a community sample and referals to a community service. International Journal of Geriatric Psychiatry 1997;12:513-518.

9. Verhey FRJ, Visser PJ. Phenomenology of depression in dementia. International Psychogeriatrics 2000;12(Suppl.1):129-134.

10. Chen P, Ganguli M, Mulsant BH, DeKosky ST. The temporal relationship between depressive symptoms and dementia: a community-based prospective study Arch Gen Psychiatry 1999;56:261-266.

11. Molloy DW, Alemayehu E, Roberts R. Reliability of a standardised Mini-mental State Examination compared to the traditional Mini-mental State Examination. American Journal of Psychiatry 1991;148:102-105.

12. Aarsland D, Tandberg E, Larsen JP, Cummings JL Frequency of dementia in Parkinson disease. Arch Neurol 1996 Jun;53(6):538-42.

13. McKeith I, Del Ser T, Spano P, Emre M, Wesnes K. Efficacy of rivastigmine in dementia with Lewy Body: a randomized, double-blind, placebo-controlled international study. Lancet 2000 Dec 16; 356(9247):2031-6

Other Reading

Monteiro IM, Stefanie RA, Boksay I, Reisberg B. New and promising modalities for assessment of behavioral and psychological symptoms of dementia. International Psychogeriatrics 2000;12[Suppl. 1]:175-178.

Sunderland T. Cholinergic contributions to behavioural disturbances in Alzheimer's disease. Internationall Psychogeriatrics 2000;12[Suppl. 1];231-235.

Mc Khann G, Drachman D, Folstein M, Katzman R, Price D, Stadlan E. Clinical diagnosis of Alzheimer's disease: Report of the NINCDS-ADRDA work group under the auspices of the Department of Health and Human Services Task Force on Alzheimer's Disease. Neurology 1984;34:939-944.

Bolla LR, Filley CM, Palmer RM. Dementia DDx. Office diagnosis of the four major types of dementia. Geriatrics 2000;55:34-37, 41-42, 45-46.

CHAPTER 5

1. Molloy DW, McIlroy WE, Guyatt GH, Lever JA. Validity and reliability of the Dysfunctional Behavioural Rating Instrument. Acta Psychiatr Scand 1991;84:103-106.

2. Molloy DW, Alemayehu E, Roberts R. Reliability of a standardised Mini-mental State Examination compared to the traditional Mini-mental State Examination. American Journal of Psychiatry 1991;148:102-105.

3. Yesavage JA, Brink TL, Rose TL, Lum O, Huang V, Adey M, Leirer O. Development of a geriatric depression screening scale: a preliminary report. Journal of Psychiatric Research 1983;17:37-49.

4. Van marwijk HW, Wallace P, De Bock GH, Hermans J, Kaptein AA, Mulder JD. Evaluation of the feasibility, reliability and diagnostic value of shortened versions of the geriatric depression scale. British Journal of General Practice, 1195;45:195-199.

5. D'Ath P, Katona P, Mullan E, et al. Screening, detection and management of depression in elderly primary care attenders. 1, The acceptability and performance of the 15-time geriatric depression scale (GDS 15) and the development of short versions. Fam Pract 1994;11:260-266.

6. Zarit SH, Reever KE, Bach-Paterson J. Relatives of the impaired elderly: correlates of feeling of burden. The Gerontologist 1980 ;20:649-55.

CHAPTER 6

1. Mittleman MS, Ferris SH, Shulman E, Steinberg G, Levin B. A family intervention to delay nursing home placement of patients with Alzheimer's disease. A randomized controlled trial. Journal of the American Medical Association 1996;276:1725-1731.

2. Brodaty H, McGilchrist C, Harris L, Peters KE. Time until institutionalisation and death in patients with dementia. Role of the caregiver training and risk factors. Archives of Neurology 1993;50:643-650.

3. Mittelman MS. Effect of support and councelling on caregiver of patients with Alzheimer's disease. International Psychogeriatrics 2000;12[Suppl. 1]:341-346.

4. Cohen-Mansfield J. Use of patient characteristics to determine nonpharmacological interventions for behavioral and psychological symptoms of dementia. International Psychogeriatrics 2000;12[Suppl. 1]:373-380.

5. Burgio LD, Fisher SE. Application of psychosocial interventions for treating behavioral and psychological symptoms of dementia. International Psychogeriatrics 2000;12[Suppl. 1]:351-358.

6. Opie J, Rosewarne R, O'Connor DW. The efficacy of psychosocial approaches to behaviour disorders in dementia: a systematic literature review. Aust N Z J Psychiatry 1999;33:789-799.

7. Gerdner LA. Music, Art, Recreational Therapies in the Treatment of Behavioral and Psychological Symptoms of Dementia. International Psychogeriatrics 2000;12[Suppl. 1]:359-366.

8. Spector A, Davies S, Woods B, Orrell M. Reality orietation for dementia: a systematic review of the evidence of effectiveness from randomised controlled trials. Gerontologist

2000;40:206-212.

9. Wettstein A, Hanhart U. Milieu Therapy for patients with dementia. Appropriate, regular stimulation by pleasant experiences. Schweiz Rundsch Med Prax 2000;89:281-286.

10. Sloane PD, Mitchell CM, Preisser JS, Phillips C, Commander C, Burker E. Environmental correlates of resident agitation in Alzheimer's disease special care units. J Am Geriatr Soc 1998;46:862-869.

11. Mintzer JE, Lewis L, Pennypaker L, Simpson W, Bachman D, Wohlreich G, Meeks A, Hunt S, Sampson R. Behavioral Intensive Care Units (BICU): a new concept in the management of acute agitated behavior in elderly demented patients. Gerontologist 1993;33:801-806.

13. Malaquin-Pavan E. Therapeutic benefit of touch-massage in the overall management of demented elderly. Rech Soins Infirm 1997:11-66.

14. Van Someren EJ, Swaab DF, Colenda CC, Cohen W, McCall WV, Rosenquist PB. Bright light therapy: improved sensitivity to its effects on rest-activity rhythms in Alzheimer patients by application of nonparametric methods. Chronobiol Int 1999;16:505-518.

15. Devereaux MA. The effects of individualised music on cognitively impaired nursing home residents exhibiting agitation. Unpublished master's thesis, College of St. Catherine, St Paul, MN. 1997.

16. Goddaer J, Abraham IL. Effects of relaxing music on agitation during meals among nursing home residents with severe cognitive impairment. Archives of Psychiatric Nursing 1994;8:150-158.

17. Tavormina CE. Embracing the Eden Alternative in Longterm care environments. *Geriatr Nurs* 1999 May-jun;20(3):158-61

18.Churchill M, Safaoui J, McCabe BW, Baun MM. Using a therapy dog to alleviate the agitation and desocialization of people with Alzheimer's disease. J Psychosoc Nurs Ment Health Serv 1999;37:16-22.

CHAPTER 7

1. Devanand DP. Conventional Neuroleptics in dementia. International Psychogeriatrics 2000;12[Suppl. 1]: 253-261.

2. Stoppe G, Brandt CA, Staedt JH. Behavioural problems associated with dementia: the role of newer antipsychotics. Drugs & Aging 1999;14:41-54.

3. Barnes R, Veith R, Okimoto J, Raskind M, Gumbrecht G. Efficacy of antipsychotic medications in behaviourally disturbed dementia patients. Am Journ of Psy 1982;139:1170-1174

4. Hamilton L, Bennett J. Acetophenazine for hyperactive geriatric patients. Geriatrics 1962;17:596-601.

5. Petrie W, Ban T, Berney S, Fujimori M, Guy W, Ragheb M et al. Loxepine in psychogeriatrics: A placebo and standard controlled clinical investigation. Journal of Clinical Psychopharmacology. 1982;2:122-126.

6. Avron J, Monane M, Everitt DE, Beers MH, Fields D. Clinical assessment of extrapyramidal signs in nursing home patients given antipsychotic medication. Archives of Internal Medicine 1994;154:1113-1117.

7. Jeste DV, Larco JP, Bailey A, Rockwell E, Harris MJ, Caligiuri MP. Lower incidence of tardive dyskinesia with risperidone compared with haloperidol in older patients. Journal of the American Geriatrics Society 1999;47:716-719.

8. Barton Frenchman I, Prince T. Clinical experience with risperidone, haloperidol and thioridazine for dementia-associated behavioral disturbances. International Psychogeriatrics 1997;9:431-435.

9. Caryle W, Anclii RJ, Sheldon L. Aggression in the demented patient: a double blind study of loxapine versus haloperidol. Int

Clin Psychopharmaclo 1993;8:103-108.

10. Katz IR, Jeste DV, Minter JE, Clyde C, Napolitano J, Brecher M. Comparison of risperidone and placebo for psychosis and behavioral distubances associated with dementia: a randomized, doubled-blind trial. Risperidone Study Group. Journal of Clinical Psychiatry 1999;60:107-115.

11. De Deyn P, Rabheru K, Rasmussen A, Bocksberger J, Dautzenberg P, Eriksson S et al. A randomized trial of risperidone, placebo and haloperidol for behaviour symptoms of dementia. Neurology 1999;53:946-955.

12. McManus D, Arvanitis L, Kowalcyk B. Quetiapine, a novel antipsychotic: experience in elderly patients with psychotic disorders. Journal of Clinical Psychiatry 1999;60:292-298.

13. Street JS, Clark WS, Gannon KS, Cummings JL, Bymaster FP et al. Olanzepine treatment of psychotic and behavioural symptoms in patients with Alzheimer's disease in nursing home care facilities: a double-blind, randomised, placebo-controlled trial. The HGEU Study Group. *Arch Gen Psychiatry* 2000 Oct;57(10):968-76.

14. Sultzer D, Gray KF, Gunay I. A double-blind comparison of trazodone and haloperidol for treatment of agitation in patients with dementia. American Journal of Geriatric Psychiatry 1997;5:60-69.

15. Swartz JR, Miller BL, Lesser IM, Darby AL. Frontotemporal dementia: treatment response to serotonin selective reuptake inhibitors. J Clin Psychiatry 1997;58:212-216.

16. Nyth AL, Gottfries CG. The clinical efficacy of citalopram in the treatment of emotional disturbances in dementia disorders. A nordic multi-center study. Br J Psychiatry 1990;157:894-901.

17. Sultzer DL. Selective serotonin reuptake inhibitors and trazadone for the treatment of depression, psychosis and behavioral symptoms in patients with dementia. International Psychogeriatrics 2000;12[Suppl. 1]:245-251.

18. Allain H, Schuck S, Bentue-Ferrer D, Bourin M, Vercelletto M et al. Anxiolytics in the treatment of Behavioural and Psychological Symptoms of Dementia. . International Psychogeriatrics 2000;12[Suppl. 1]:281-289.

19. Christensen DB, Benfield WR. Alprazolam as an alternative to low-dose haloperidol in older, cognitively impaired nursing facility patients. J Am Geriatr Soc 1998;46:620-625.

20. Grossman F. A review of anticonvulsants in treating agitated demented elderly patients. Pharmacotherapy 1998;18:600-606.

21. Tariot PN, Erb R, Leibovici A. Carbamazepine treatment of agitation in nursing home patients with dementia: a preliminary study. American Journal of Geriatric Psychiatry 1994;42;1160-1166.

22. Tariot P, Erb R, Podgorski C, Patel S, Jakimovich L et al. Efficacy and tolerability of carbamazepine for agitation and aggression in dementia. American Journal of Psychiatry 1998;155:54-61.

23. Mellow A, Solano-Lopez C, Davis S. Sodium valproate in the treatment of behavioral disturbance in dementia. Journal of Geriatric Psychiatry & Neurology 1993;6:205-209.

24. Hermann N. Valporic acid treatment of agitation in dementia. Canadian Journal of Psychiatry-Revue Canadienne de Psychiatrie 1998;43:69-72.

25. Lindenmayer JP, Kotsaftis A. Use of sodium valproate in violent and aggressive behaviors: a critical review. J Clin Psychiatry 2000;61:123-8.

26. Goad D, Davis C, Liem P, Fuselier C, McCormack J, Olssen K. The use of selegiline in Alzheimer's patients with behavior problems. Journal of Clinical Psychiatry 1991;52:342-345.

27. Lawlor BA, Radcliffe J, Molchan SE. A pilot placebo controlled study of trazodone and buspirone in Alzheimer's disease. International Journal of Geriatric Psychiatry 1994;9:55-59.

28. Cummings JL, Gorman DG, Shapira J. Physostigmine ameliorates the delusions of Alzheimer's disease. Biol Psychiatry 1993;33:536-541.

29. Cummings JL. Cholinseterase inhibitors: A new class of psychotropic compounds. Am J Psychiatry 2000;157:4-15.

30. Reisberg B, Borenstein J, Salob SP, Ferris SH, Franssen E, Georgotas A. Behavioural symptoms in Alzheimer's disease:phenomenology and treatment. *Journal of Clinical Psychiatry.* 1987;48 (suppl 5):9-15.

31. Barak Y, Wittenberg N, Noar S, Kutzut D, Weizman A. Clozapine in elderly psychiatric patients: tolerability, safety, and efficacy. *Compr Psychiatry* 1999 Jul-Aug;40(4):320-5.

32. Trosch RM, Friedman JH, Lannon MC, Pahwa R, Smith D, et al. Clozapine use in Parkinson's disease: a retrospective analysis of a large multicentered clinical experience. *Mov Disord* 1998 May;13(3):377-82

33. Amadeo M Anti-androgen treatment for aggressivity in men suffering from dementia. J Geriatr Psychiatry Neurol 1996 Jul;9(3):142-5

34. Weiler PG, Mungas D, Bernick C. Propranolol for the control of disruptive behaviour in senile dementia. J Geriatr Psychiatry Neurol 1998 1:226-230

35. Greendyke RM, Kanter DR. Therapeutic effects of pindolol on behavoural disturbances associated with organic brain disorders:Adouble blind study.J Clin Psychiatry 1986 47(8):423-427.

36. Sakauye KM, Camp CJ, Ford PA. Effects of buspirone on agitation associated with dementia. 1993 Am J Geriatr Psychiatry 1(1):82-84.

37. Tran PV, Hamilton SH, Kuntz AJ, Potvin JH, Anderson SW. Double-blind comparison of olanzapine versus risperidone in the treatment of schizophrenia and other psychotic disorders. J Clin Psychopharmacol 1997;17(5):407-418

38. McKeith I, Del Ser T, Spano P, Emre M, Wesnes K. Efficacy of rivastigmine in dementia with Lewy Body: a randomized, double-blind, placebo-controlled international study. Lancet 2000 Dec 16; 356(9247):2031-6.

REFERENCES

Other Reading

Jeste DV, Rockwell E, Harris MJ, Lohr JB, Lacro J. Conventional vs. newer antipsychotics in the elderly patients Am J Geriatric Psychiatry 1999;7:70-76.

Maixner S, Mellow A, Tandon R. The efficacy, safety and tolerability of antipsychotics in the elderly. Journal of Clinical Psychiatry 1996;60[Suppl. 8]:29-41.

Tariot P, Gaile SE, Castelli NA, Thorsteinsson AP. Treatment of agitation in dementia. New Directions for Mental Health Services 1997:109-123.

American Psychiatric Association. Practice guideline for the treatment of patients with Alzheimer's disease and other dementias of late life. American Journal of Psychiatry 1997;154[Suppl. 5]:1-39.

Tariot P, Schneider L, Katz I. Anticonvulsant and other non-neuroleptic treatment of agitation in dementia. Journal of Geriatric Psychiatry & Neurology 1995;8[Suppl. 1]:S28-S39.

Olanzapine reduces psychotic symptoms and behavioural disturbances asssociated with Alzheimer's disease. London,UK:12th Congress of the European College of Neuropsychopharmacology, 1999.

Mazure CM, Druss BG, Cellar JS. Valproate treatment of older psychotic patients with organic mental syndromes and behavioral dyscontrol.Journal of the American Geriatrics Society 1992;40:914-916.

Simpson D, Foster D. Improvement in organically disturbed behaviour with trazodone treatment. Journal of Clinical Psychiatry 1986;47:191-193.

Schneider LS, Sobin PB. Non-neuroleptic medications in the management of agitation in Alzheimer's disease and other dementia: a selective review. International Journal of Geriatric Psychiatry 1991;6:691-701.

Tariot PN, Cohen RM, Sunderland T. L-Deprenyl in Alzheimer's disease: preliminary evidence for behavioral change with monoamino oxidase B inhibition. Archives of General Psychiatry 1987;44:427-433.

Petrie W, Ban T, Berney S, Fujimori M, Guy W, Ragheb M et al.Loxapine in psychogeriatrics: A placebo-and standard-controlled clinical investigation. Journal of Clinical Psychopharmacology 1982;2:122-126.

Owens D. Extrapyramidal side effects and tolerability of risperidone: A review. Journal of Clinical Psychiatry 1994;55[Suppl. 5]:29S-35S.

Caliguiri M, Lacro J, Jeste D. Incidence and predictors of drug-induced parkinsonisim in older psychiatric patients treated with very low doses of neuroleptics. Journal of Clinical Psychopharmacology 1999;19:322-328.

Lee H, Conney J Lawlor B. The use of risperidone an atypical neuroleptic in lewy body disease. International Journal of Geriatric Psychiatry 1994;9:415-417.
Magnuson T, Keller B, Burke W. Extrapyramidal side effects in a patient treated with risperidone plus donepezil. American Journal of Psychiatry 1998;155:1458-1459.

CHAPTER 8

1. Mendez MF, Perryman KM, Miller BL, Swartz JR, Cummings. Compulsive behaviours as presenting symptoms of frontotemporal dementia. J Geriatr Psychiatry Neurol 1997 Oct;10(4):154-7

2. Casby JA, Holm MB. The effect of music on repetitive disruptive vocalizations of persons with dementia. Am J Occup Ther 1994;48:883-889.

3. Pulman J, Yassa R, Ananth J. Clomipramine treatment of repetitive behavior. Can J Psychiatry 1984;29:254-255.

4. Raskind MA. Evaluation and management of aggressive behavior in the elderly demented patients. J Clin Psychiatry 1999;60[Suppl. 15]:45-49.

5. Lyketsos CG, Steele C, Galik E, Rosenblatt A, Steinberg M. Physical aggression in dementia patients and it's relationship with depression Am J Psychiatry 1999 Jan ;156(1):66-71.

6. Taylor JL, Friedman L, Sheikh J, Yesavage JA. Assessment and management of "Sundowning" phenomena. Semin Clin Neuropsychiatry 1997;2:113-122.

7. Hess CW. Sleep disorders and dementia. Schweiz Rundsch Med Prax 1997;86:1343-1349.

8. Mullan E, Katona C, Bellew M. Patterns of sleep disorders and sedative hypnotic use in seniors. Drugs Aging 1994;5:49-58.

9. Starkstein SE Migliorelli R Manes F Teson A Petracca G The prevalance and clinical correlates of apathy and irritability in Alzheimer's disease European Journal of Neurology 1995 ;2:540-546.

10. Starkstein SE. Apathy and Withdrawal. International Psychogeriatrics 2000;Vol 12[Suppl. 1]:35-137.

11. Keene J, Hope T. Natural history of hyperphagia and other eating changes in dementia. Int J Geritr Psychiatry 1998;13:700-706.

12. Volicier L, Stelly M, Morris J, McLaughlin J, Volicer BJ. Effects of dronabinol on anorexxia and disturbed behaviour in patients with Alzheimer's disease. Int J Geriatr Psychiatry 1997Sep;12(9):913-9

13. Keene JM, Hope T. Hyperphagia in dementia: 1. The use of an objective and reliable method for measuring hyperphagia in people with dementia. Appetite 1997;28:151-65.

14. Keene JM, Hope T. Hyperphagia in dementia: 2. Food choices and their macronutrient contents in hyperphagia, dementia and ageing. Appetite 1997;28:167-175.

15. Holroyd S, Sheldon-Keller A. A study of visual hallucinations in Alzheimer's disease. American Journal of Geriatric Psychiatry ;3:198-205.

16. Holroyd S. Hallucinations and Delusions in Dementia. International Psychogeriatrics 2000;12[Suppl. 1]:113-117.

17. Bassiony MM, Steinberg MS, Warren A, Rosenblatt A, Baker AS, Lyketsos CG. Delusions and hallucinations in Alzheimer's disease: prevalence and clinical correlates. Int J Geriatr Psychiatry 2000;15:99-107.

18. Wragg RE, Jeste DV. Overview of depression and psychosis in Alzheimer's disease. American Journal of Psychiatry 1989;146:577-587.

19. Logsdon RG, Teri L, McCurry SM, Gibbons LE, Kukall WA, Larson EB. Wandering: a significant problem among community-residing individuals with Alzheimer's disease. J

Gerontol B Psychol Sci Sci 1998 Sep;53(5):p294-9

20. Klein DA, Steinberg M, Galik E, Steele C, Sheppard JM et al . Wandering behaviour in community –residing persons with dementia. Int J Geriatr Psychiatry 1999 Apr;14(4):272-9.

21. Holmberg SK A walking program for wanderers: volunteer training and development of an evening walker's group. Geriatr Nurs. 1997 Jul-Aug;18(4):160-5.

22. Hwang JP, Tsai SJ, Yang CH, Liu KM, Lirng JF Hoarding behavior in dementia. A preliminary report. Am J Geriatr Psychiatry 1998 Fall;6(4):285-9

23. Tariot PN. Treatment of agitation in dementia. J Clin Psychiatry 1999;60 [suppl8]:11-20.

Other Reading

Endale, Genda Y, Rummans T. Pain: cause of agitation in elderly individuals with dementia. American Journal of Psychiatry 1999;156:1662-1663.

Bourgeois MS, Burgio LD, Schulz R, Beach S, Palmer B. Modifying repetitive verbalizations of community-dwelling patients with AD. Gerontologist 1997;37:30-39.

Hope T, Tilling KM, Gedling K, Keene JM, Cooper D, Fairburn CG. The structure of wandering in dementia. International Journal of Geriatric Psychiatry 1994;9:149-155.

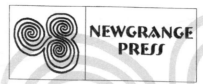

P U B L I C A T I O N S

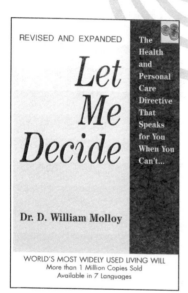

REVISED AND EXPANDED

Let Me Decide

The Health and Personal Care Directive That Speaks for You When You Can't...

Dr. D. William Molloy

WORLD'S MOST WIDELY USED LIVING WILL
More than 1 Million Copies Sold
Available in 7 Languages

- Gives each individual the opportunity to choose different levels of treatment according to his or her wishes.

- Helps relieve family and friends of responsibility for decisions in a time of crisis.

- Guides health care practitioners in making vital decisions when family members are unavailable.

- Has received enthusiastic support from a wide variety of individuals and groups including doctors, patients, social workers, lawyers, clergy and advocates for the elderly and the disabled.

THE *LET ME DECIDE* PROGRAM

Through age, illness or accident, people may lose their capacity to understand the nature and consequences of proposed health and personal care decisions. These decisions then fall to families, friends and physicians who may not be aware of the patient's wishes and intent. The health care directive contained in this booklet lets you plan your own future health and personal care in advance. It makes sure your wishes will be known, when you no longer can understand your options or communicate your choices to others. Developed over many years of research and consultation, the *Let Me Decide* health and personal care directive.

Continued on next page

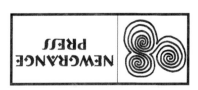

NEWGRANGE PRESS

FOR MORE INFORMATION OR TO ORDER

Newgrange Press (Canada)
428 Orkney Road, RR1 Troy, Ontario, Canada L0R 2B0
Tel: (905) 628-0354 Fax: (905) 628-4901
E-mail: idecide@netcom.ca
Website: www.newgrangepress.com

Newgrange Press (U.S.A.)
301 Highland Avenue
Winchester, MA 01890
telephone/fax: 781.729.8981
E-mail: jamesmcinerny@hotmail.com

Newgrange Press (Ireland)
The Stables, Woodstown, Waterford, Ireland
Tel: 353-51-870152 Fax: 353-51-871214

Newgrange Press (Australia)
P.O. Box 7077 Shenton Park, W. Australia 6008
Tel: 08-9346-8107 Fax:08-9346 8232
E-mail: clarnett@medeserv.com.au

Newgrange Press (Japan)
100-1, Kashiyama, Habikino, Osaka (583-0886) Japan
Tel: 81729-542000 Fax: 81-729-547560

Newgrange Press (Austria)
Willersdorferstrasse 6
A-8061 St. Radegund Austria
Tel: 0043-3132-3472 Fax: 0043-3132-3472-15

*Payment can be made by cheque or money order payable to
"Newgrange Press" Books will be mailed within 7 days of payment.*

NEWGRANGE PRESS ORDER FORM

Let Me Decide (LMD) Booklets	Price	Qty
English	$10.00	
French	$10.00	
German	$15.00	
Italian	$10.00	
Japanese	$15.00	
Spanish	$10.00	
Swedish	$15.00	
LMD Audio Tape/Talking Book	$15.00	
LMD Single Videos (English ○ French ○)		
My Health Care - I Decide	$30.00	
My Health Care - Understanding My Choices	$30.00	
My Health Care - Filling out the Directive	$30.00	
Video Series (set of 3) (English ○ French ○)	$90.00	
LMD Bulk/Directive/forms		
Personal	$1.00ea.	
Next-of-Kin	$1.00ea.	
LMD "The Works" complete package includes:	$150.00	
3 Videos (English ○ French ○)		
1 Set of Slides		
1 Let Me Decide Book (English, French, German, Spanish, Italian Research Publications)		
SADAS Workbooks (Set of 4)	$50.00 ea	
SADAS Training Manual	$20.00	
Capacity to Decide	$24.00	
How Do you Say? (Italian ver. Com Si Dice)	$14.00	
Standardized Mini Mental State Exam. (SMMSE)	$5.00	
SMMSE User's Guide	$10.00	
Visions and Voices... The Nurse Practitioner Today	$20.00	
Nurse Practitioners... The Catalyst of Change	$24.00	
Let Me Pass Gently	$29.95	
Set Me Free	$10.00	
Dysfunctional Behaviour in Dementia: A Clinician's Guide	$15.00	
Total of Order *Please add 7% GST on Canadian orders and sales tax where applicable on US orders*		
Postage & Handling, 15% (or minimum of $2.50) on total order only		
GRAND TOTAL:		

HOW DO YOU SAY?
(Italian Version Com Si Dice)
Dr. D. W. Molloy and Dr. S. Salama

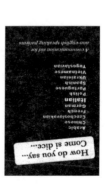

Practical, user friendly communication aid for health care workers and Italian patients. Contains sections on general conversation, personal needs, medical terms, pictionary and dictionary.

TRAIN THE TRAINER WORKSHOP

The LET ME DECIDE workshop is a two-day seminar which teaches you to effectively implement advance health care directives in long term care, acute care institutions, and in the community using a systematic well-planned approach.

This workshop will focus upon:

Introduction to directives
Completing Directives
How to use Directives in Your Organization

All participants will receive a complete educational package containing the following:

- A comprehensive workshop reference manual.
- The *LET ME DECIDE* booklet and directive insert.
- Published articles and other reading material on the directive.
- Train the Trainer Certificate

Cost of two-day Workshop $500.00 per person
enrollment limited
maximum 25 participants

VISIT OUR WEB SITE FOR MORE DETAILS!

NURSE PRACTITIONERS... THE CATALYST OF CHANGE
Christine Patterson (Editor)

A new nurse practitioner book, complementary to Visions and Voices. Both books are timely and make a significant contribution to outlining how nursing organized itself to realize a vision.

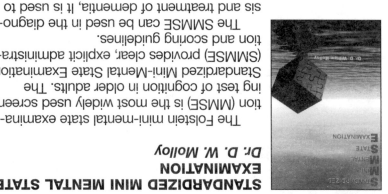

STANDARDIZED MINI MENTAL STATE EXAMINATION
Dr. D. W. Molloy

The Folstein mini-mental state examination (MMSE) is the most widely used screening test of cognition in older adults. The Standardized Mini-Mental State Examination (SMMSE) provides clear, explicit administration and scoring guidelines.

The SMMSE can be used in the diagnosis and treatment of dementia. It is used to stage the disease, differentiate between the different dementias and assess response to treatment.

STANDARDIZED MINI MENTAL STATE EXAMINATION: A USER'S GUIDE
Dr. D. W. Molloy and Dr. Roger Clarnette

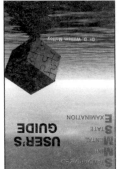

This short booklet contains a standardized version of the Standardized Mini-Mental State Examination (SMMSE) and describes how this short test can be used to diagnose and treat cognitive impairment in older adults. This book describes how the SMMSE is used to stage dementia, assess treatment and develop care plans.

The pattern changes on the SMMSE provide valuable clues to the cause of cognitive impairment. This short booklet is packed with practical clinical tips, diagnostic aids, tables and figures.

VISIONS AND VOICES ...
THE NURSE PRACTITIONER TODAY
Christine Patterson (Editor)

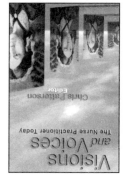

Visions and Voices: The Nurse Practitioner Today is a comprehensive overview of the political, economic and social factors that influence advanced practice role of nurses. In this book, contributors from different organizations outline the political process, educational challenges and legal implications of advance practice.

Nurse practitioners discuss their roles and the problems faced in role development. Physicians relate their experiences working with nurse practitioners in different primary, secondary and tertiary care settings. This book is a unique, detailed account of the challenges faced by professional nursing as it redefines its role in health care.

LET ME PASS GENTLY

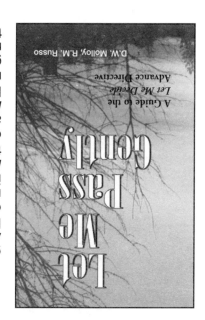

This is a comprehensive guide to the *Let Me Decide* "Advance Directive Program. This book describes the legal, clinical, ethical, spiritual, social and economic issues with the use of *Let Me Decide* program in different settings and different countries. It contains a wealth of information about advance directives and the *Let Me Decide* program. "Let Me Pass Gently" provides the instruments developed for the program, policies, case histories, terminology and over thirty publications on Let Me Decide.

Let Me Decide is available in French, German, Italian, Japanese, Spanish and Swedish. Let Me Decide is a complete health care program with three videos in English and French.

1) My Health Care - I Decide
2) My Health Care - Understanding My Choices
3) My Health Care - Filling out the Directive

"Train the Trainer" Workshops and lectures are available on request.

CAPACITY TO DECIDE
Dr. D. W. Molloy Dr. P. Darzins, Dr. Strang

Capacity to Decide is a short, comprehensive book which describes a new six step capacity assessment that measures decision-specific capacity, with clear instructions on its use. This book describes how this new assessment process can be applied to measure capacity for:

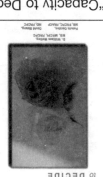

- personal care
- Wills and Power of Attorney
- health care
- driving
- property and finances
- sexuality and intimacy
- advance directives

"Capacity to Decide" is a practical guide and invaluable tool for health care workers, members of the legal profession and anyone who needs to measure capacity in patients or clients.

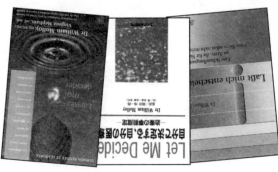